THE NEW
LOW-CARB DIET
COOKBOOK

Groundbreaking recipes for healthy, long-term weight loss

Laura Lamont

dbp

DUNCAN BAIRD PUBLISHERS

LONDON

The New Low-Carb Diet Cookbook
Laura Lamont

First published in the United Kingdom and Ireland
in 2014 by Duncan Baird Publishers, an imprint of
Watkins Publishing Limited
PO Box 883, Oxford, OX1 9PL

A member of Osprey Group
enquiries@dbp.co.uk

Publisher: Grace Cheetham
Editor: Wendy Hobson
Managing Designer: Suzanne Tuhrim
Commissioned Photography: Toby Scott, except on pages
8, 57, 93, 101 and 153 by Noel Murphy
Food Stylists: Jayne Cross, except on pages 95, 142, 147, 149,
155 and 157 by Jennie Shapter and on pages 8, 57, 93, 101
and 153 by Rebecca Rauter
Prop Stylist: Wei Tang
Production: Uzma Taj

A CIP record for this book is available from the British Library

ISBN: 978-1-84899-112-5

10 9 8 7 6 5 4 3 2 1

Typeset in Myriad Pro and Roboto
Colour reproduction by PDQ, UK
Printed in China

Notes on the Recipes

- Unless otherwise stated:
- Use medium eggs, fruit and vegetables
- Use fresh ingredients, including herbs and spices
- Do not mix metric and imperial measurements
  1 tsp = 5ml   1 tbsp = 15ml   1 cup = 250ml

Publisher's Note

While every care has been taken in compiling the recipes for
this book, Watkins Publishing Limited, or any other persons
who have been involved in working on this publication,
cannot accept responsibility for any errors or omissions,
inadvertent or not, that may be found in the recipes or text,
nor for any problems that may arise as a result of preparing
one of these recipes. If you are pregnant or breastfeeding or
have any special dietary requirements or medical conditions,
it is advisable to consult a medical professional before
following any of the recipes contained in this book.

CONTENTS

INTRODUCTION

Are you fed up with fasting? Crabby from your crash diet? And tired of being on a different diet plan every month? Are you looking for an easy, fresh, new approach to losing weight quickly and maintaining it for life, while being able to include your whole family in your improved healthy lifestyle at the same time? Well, I know from personal experience exactly what that feels like. I also know from my experience as a qualified nutritional therapist and diet coach exactly what to do about it. The crucial factor is what I believe to be the missing link in the traditional way of low-carb and low-fat dieting that seems to have taken centre stage in the dieting world.

Once I had qualified as a nutritional therapist, I decided to focus all my attention on weight loss, as this single factor is such a huge trigger to so many other health problems that we have today. As the director of a diet coaching clinic, I saw many different people with the same weight issues and battles. After seeing endless clients in the clinic who had been struggling with yo-yo dieting, I began to notice a strong correlation between carbohydrate addiction and the inability to stick to a weight-loss programme. I also noticed that every one of these clients had that same old-school understanding that in order to lose weight you had to cut down on fat. Because fat is high in calories, cutting it out of the diet generally leaves you hungry, and so you fill up on starchy carbohydrates like bread, pasta and potatoes as well as oodles of vegetables and fruit. The latter may be low in fat and full of healthy nutrients, but they are also extremely high in sugar and refined carbohydrate – both of which will cause you to put on weight, not lose it. So I found that this old-fashioned way of dieting would potentially give good results in the short term, because it did reduce the calorie intake, but as a long-term strategy, it was just not sustainable. The downside of this kind of weight-loss programme is that it also leads to very unstable blood sugar levels, which inevitably result in energy fluctuations and cravings for more carbohydrates. And, of course, that means you don't stick to the diet.

These ingrained, old-fashioned ideas of weight loss combined with the huge numbers of low-fat and low-calorie but high-sugar products available today have really played havoc with people's blood sugar levels and left them feeling hungry and out of control. This left me pondering. Could the low-fat craze of the 1950s and the array of low-fat, half-fat, reduced-fat and low-calorie foods that have come on to the market be the trigger for the sudden rise in obesity and diabetes that followed?

So I devised a plan for a new version of a simple carbohydrate-controlled diet. Even if you are trying to lose weight, carbohydrates are still a valuable source of energy but what we want are the complex carbs that release their energy slowly, not the simple carbs that give you a sugar rush followed by a dip, so my programme was structured so that carbohydrates were not cut out completely, but complex carbs were allowed in small quantities, with the main hit of carbohydrate being at breakfast. This creates a slow release of sugar into the blood stream, giving you plenty of energy, but avoiding the energy crash later.

As well as being centred around the carbohydrate-control principle, this diet is also calorie controlled, which is always a very important element of any diet for weight loss. But don't worry, as you won't be doing any calorie counting yourself if you follow this book. This has all been done for you.

Once I had established the success of my low-carb diet, I began implementing the addition of fats into the diet, either combined with or in place of carbohydrates and sugars, and I monitored the effect on my clients that this had on cravings and hunger levels. The results were astonishing in both weight loss and improvement in many health conditions. And the best thing was that the cravings went away completely, meaning that my clients were actually able to stick to the plan long term, signalling the end of their yo-yo dieting nightmares for ever!

The only problem that I encountered with my clients on this diet was that they seemed to hit a plateau of weight loss after a few months on the plan. This is very common in weight loss as your body naturally starts to adjust to the new, lower calorie intake. But the good news is that getting stuck on this plateau is easily prevented with the addition of a tasty treat – how good is that? This is why you can enjoy a decadent dessert once a week on this plan without the slightest feeling of guilt because this regular calorie surge will prevent your body hitting this plateau and stalling your successful weight loss.

While a high-fat diet may seem controversial, there are actually scores of current research papers showing this to be a safe and very effective way to lose weight. Despite that, this new concept in dieting and weight loss just isn't getting out into public awareness fast enough to benefit all the people who are struggling to achieve and maintain a healthy weight in the long term. This book aims to change that. All fingers point to this low-carb, high-fat diet being the magic key to getting to grips with the obesity epidemic, and even providing a possible answer to the diabetes problem that is being fuelled by the low-fat, high-carbohydrate diet industry that we have today. From this new understanding and improved way of thinking, I have created my New Low-Carb Diet in order to try and put this right for the many people who are suffering from the adverse effects of traditional diets.

CHAPTER 1
THE NEW LOW-CARB DIET

This is a diet designed to help you lose weight and maintain a healthy weight. The plan is simple, straightforward and it works – I know this because it is the original plan I use in my clinic to successfully treat clients with obesity.

So what can it help you to achieve?

- Shed at least 900g/2lb a week while dieting, losing it mainly from your waist
- Stop yo-yo dieting: constantly losing weight, then putting it back on
- Boost your metabolism and increase your energy
- Curb your cravings for sugar-laden junk foods and heavy carbohydrate-based meals
- Improve your blood sugar stability
- Lower cholesterol levels and blood pressure

- Even out mood swings
- Improve your skin
- Give you better sleep patterns
- Teach you portion control and strengthen your willpower
- Establish a pattern for healthy eating for life

The plan is based on low-carbohydrate, high-fat, high-protein principles, so you choose foods in the right ratios and the right quantities. But it also incorporates other scientifically proven findings that help speed up weight loss.

So, if you are finally ready to stop yo-yo dieting and end that binge-diet cycle for ever, let's get started on the road to a new, slimmer, happier you!

THE PLAN & THE BENEFITS

The New Low-Carb Diet is tried and tested, easy to follow and really works. It involves no calorie counting or point scoring. All you do is choose from the recipes in the appropriate section of the book, or construct your meals by choosing the right proportions from several different colour groups.

- **Free** Contains foods you can eat in any quantity.
- **Blue** Comprises protein foods that are essential for building and repairing the body's cells.
- **Yellow** Includes all the fats, such as milk, butter, oil and cream.
- **Red** Contains the complex carbohydrates that give you slow-release energy.
- **Green** Encompasses all the vegetables.

This gives you a broad choice of food options for each meal and snack, and allows for plenty of variation and choice. At the same time, this method will teach you about which choices you should be making when it comes to staple foods such as bread, cereals and rice, as well as teaching you about portion control. This will soon become so automatic that you will start making healthy choices without thinking about it, inspiring healthy home cooking that can be shared with the whole family.

Don't miss out

No one is going to stick to a diet that doesn't offer great eating, so in this book you'll find a collection of imaginative recipes that everyone in the household will enjoy, with the added benefit that you won't need to cook something different for yourself. And once you are used to the system, you will have established your healthy-eating regime for life.

In contrast to most diet books, *The New Low-Carb Diet Cookbook* doesn't cut out any food groups or prevent you from having the occasional treat, such as chocolate, caffeine, alcohol or even a full-blown dessert. Instead, it puts you in control and gives you the option of incorporating these things into your diet, if you choose. You will be pleased to know that you can even enjoy bread daily on this diet. A portion of good, slow-release carbohydrate at breakfast really gets your energy levels off to a positive start for the day. It may surprise you to be offered the occasional indulgent dessert. Although healthier options are always encouraged, I firmly believe that by completely cutting out the special treats that we love, we are only setting ourselves up to fail. This plan helps you learn how to eat a healthy diet for ever, and a future without the occasional slice of cake is just not acceptable!

Scientifically proven

Although the plan is centred on low-carbohydrate, high-fat principles, I have also made full use of scientifically proven and highly researched findings that help speed up weight loss in different ways. These are set out in my 10 weight-loss diet tricks (see pages 22–33), all of which are incorporated into the plan and encouraged throughout.

Boosts energy levels

The big changes that you will start to notice almost immediately when you embark on the New Low-Carb Diet include a massive boost in your energy levels and an elevation in your mood. You should find that your sleep pattern is much improved, too, which will contribute to you feeling more alert and focused throughout the day. Plus there's the added bonus that your skin will tend to be clearer and more radiant.

Curbs cravings

While traditional diets can leave you hungry – with the obvious consequence that you quickly give up – this diet makes sure your body doesn't succumb to those hunger cravings. That means you are far more likely to stick to it and break the boom-and-bust cycle.

Restores balance

For some people, potential health problems or imbalances can hold them back from their weight-loss goal, making it almost impossible for them to achieve their optimum weight without them even realizing it. These problems might be anything from minor vitamin deficiencies to major digestive imbalances. Nothing is more demoralizing than trying to do things 'right' without the rewards of success, so it is important to address such issues early on. Consult your doctor for professional advice.

Helps control diabetes, cholesterol and blood pressure

As well as fast weight loss and improved health, interestingly, I have also seen my diet plan help to alleviate the symptoms of Type 2 diabetes, help to lower harmful cholesterol and – even more amazingly – lower blood pressure.

So let's find out how and why this diet plan can help you to achieve all this.

THE SCIENCE BEHIND THE DIET

If you are trying to make positive changes to your diet, you are far more likely to succeed if you stick to the principles of the plan. So this section gives you the information you need on the background to this new low-carbohydrate diet. If you actually understand the reasons why this diet works, you will feel comfortable with the plan from the outset, and start out towards your weight-loss goal with confidence and enthusiasm.

So first, let's sketch in the bigger picture.

Why low-fat diets don't work

We all know that the basics of weight loss come down to the straightforward equation of calories in and calories out. Simply put, in order to lose weight, the body has to be burning more calories than it is taking in, so that it then begins to burn calories that have been stored in the body as fat. Simple, right? Well, not quite so simple, because the huge downfall is that we just don't seem to be able to stick to this in the long term.

Why? The real reason that it is so difficult to stick to diets is that we so often turn to low-fat foods in order to reduce our calorie intake. Take fat out of our diet and we end up hungry – and then we reach for the comforting carbohydrates, because no one can stick to a diet that leaves them hungry all the time. Add to that the fact that these low-fat packaged foods come with loads of added sugar and sweeteners to make them taste better, and you find that low fat often means high calories. The consequence of that, of course, is that these low-fat/high-sugar foods then give us a massive sugar high, which triggers the release of the hormone insulin.

How does insulin work?

The role of insulin is to take excess sugar away from the blood to be stored as fat. So if you are regularly eating low-fat meals and snacks that are high in carbohydrates, you are triggering sugar highs and therefore rushes of insulin, which are inevitably followed by sugar lows. These fluctuating blood sugar levels cause your body not only to store away fat but, what's more, this insulin effect makes you feel hungry, tired and prone to both mood swings and cravings for more food. You can begin to feel like you are out of control on a never-ending rollercoaster.

Do you recognize this scenario in your diet? If you feel like a failure when it comes to dieting, this should encourage you because it may be that it is not your fault that you are finding it so hard to control your weight. It is your body's natural reaction to the sugar rollercoaster and the fault lies in the massive misinformation about dieting that so many people have accepted as fact.

How do we stop the sugar rollercoaster?

So how do we prevent this yo-yo effect? First we need to limit the carbohydrates we eat so that our bodies become fat burners rather than fat storers. Then we need to choose the right kind of carbohydrates, ditching the simple carbs, like sugar, and choosing the complex carbs, like oats. Simple carbohydrates are broken down quickly in the body, releasing energy in a burst and triggering that same release of insulin. Complex carbohydrates are broken down slowly without triggering this major insulin response.

So the first step is to avoid simple carbohydrates and sugars in our diet in order to prevent these insulin bursts, and that means avoiding too many sweet things and ditching the packaged foods that are full of simple carbohydrates. But we can still enjoy the slow-release, complex carbohydrates in the morning. Why the morning? Because that way our breakfast will do its work, gradually releasing the energy we need to keep going and to sustain our mood, making sure we remain on an even keel throughout the day without stimulating cravings for sugary snacks.

And what about fat?

It may sound counterintuitive, but it's a proven fact that we need to eat fat to burn fat. So the most important message here is to incorporate more fat in our diet – that's right, fat is actually good for weight loss because it helps to lower the impact of sugar in the blood stream. As with carbohydrates, there is more than one type of fat, and the 'good' fat is the one found in oily fish, flaxseeds and walnuts known as omega-3.

So let's look at how fat keeps us healthy and helps us lose weight and maintain a healthy weight.

- Fat helps stabilize blood sugar levels, preventing the release of insulin and thus limiting the energy stored as fat.
- Fat keeps us feeling fuller for longer because it takes a lot longer to digest than simple sugars and other carbohydrates, so makes us eat a lot less.
- Fat helps to improve leptin sensitivity, which is what I call the 'thin hormone'.

The importance of leptin

Leptin is a small but powerful hormone that has been relatively recently discovered and that has now been shown to be hugely significant in the weight-loss equation. Partly because we have not understood this important hormone for very long, it seems to have taken a back seat to insulin in our understanding of weight loss and how we apply that understanding in practice. But I believe it is just as significant to understand how leptin works as to understand how insulin works, and only when we do that will we be in a better position to explain why people find it so hard to lose weight and therefore why the obesity epidemic is ever-increasing.

Leptin is the messenger hormone that tells our brain when we feel satisfied and that we should stop eating, so it is obviously a crucial part of our diet picture. Logic might tell us that the more leptin we have circulating in the blood, the better, but unfortunately that couldn't be further from the truth. This is because it isn't a question of quantity but of quality, the key factor being how sensitive our body is to the leptin and therefore how effective our body is in making sure these vital messages reach the brain.

If we constantly over-eat, then our body reacts by releasing a continual stream of leptin into the blood. Not surprisingly, the receptors that transport it to the brain become worn out and aren't able to get the right message to the brain. If the brain doesn't get the leptin message telling it we have eaten enough, it naturally thinks we are in a state of famine. So instead of telling our body to stop eating, it does the opposite: it triggers intense hunger and cravings. Hardly what we need when we are trying to stick to a restricted diet plan! Therefore it sets off another vicious cycle that makes us put on even more weight.

But that's not the end of this amazing hormone's qualities because studies have shown that it actually makes us want to exercise more. So if you have been thinking you are just being lazy or feeling too tired to hit the gym, it could be the result of decreased leptin sensitivity. Solve that, and you could actually want to exercise – wouldn't that be great?

There's one final point in understanding why balanced levels of leptin are so important. It is well known that fat accumulation in the muscles is a major contributing factor towards insulin resistance, which is the most common first step towards Type 2 diabetes. But when leptin is working efficiently, it actually decreases the fat storage in the muscles and so can greatly improve insulin resistance and therefore reduce the potential for developing Type 2 diabetes.

Optimizing leptin efficiency

So, as an appetite suppressant, to encourage us to exercise and to reduce muscle-fat storage, we need leptin and its receptors to be working efficiently, and we can achieve that by making just a few changes to our diet. We know that leptin resistance occurs in response to high blood glucose levels, so sugary foods and drinks and refined carbohydrates are a sure fire way to a leptin disaster and are best avoided if you want to lose weight and stay healthy. Everything points in the same direction – towards cutting out refined sugars.

However, what you may not realize is that the natural sugars found in fruit can actually have the same negative effect on leptin, because the high levels of fructose – fruit sugars – can interfere with the ability of leptin to cross the blood-brain barrier, resulting in leptin resistance. We all know that fruit is good for us, low in fat and gives us a good supply of vitamins and fibre. But if we want to lose weight, we also need to limit our fruit intake because fruit is actually detrimental to weight loss because of the effect of these sugars on the effectiveness of leptin. On the other hand, increasing whole grains and green leafy vegetables in the diet is thought to improve leptin sensitivity, so including plenty of them in our diet has an added benefit.

Two final important factors in improving leptin resistance are getting enough sleep and lowering stress levels. Leptin levels naturally rise while we sleep, while when we are stressed, the body releases the hormone cortisol, which can actually inhibit healthy leptin function.

Avoiding the famine response

Interestingly, it is also believed that when we suddenly reduce our calorie intake by starting a diet plan, it actually takes a long time before the body acclimatizes to the reduced food intake. This means that our body suddenly thinks that we are going to starve and instinctively switches off leptin production to make us feel more hungry. Obviously this is not going to help us lose weight and stick to our diet plan. But don't worry, as this diet plan has a simple way of tricking the body out of this reaction: one day a week, we eat more calories. I told you it was simple! That stops the body thinking it is in a state of famine, prevents it from getting comfortable with the set level of calories and, in doing so, prevents you from hitting a plateau. So during this plan you will be having one day a week where you get to indulge in an after-dinner dessert.

LET'S GET STARTED

Now you understand the basic nutritional principles, it's time to start taking action, so let's highlight the main points in order to strengthen your confidence and determination to succeed.

Unstable blood sugar levels are the main contributor to weight gain and make weight loss a constant battle. They are also detrimental to mood and energy levels, both of which trigger comfort eating, thereby making things worse. In the long term, they can lead to all kinds of health problems.

If we eat simple, or refined, carbohydrates – like pure sugar and fruit sugars – the body doesn't need to put in any work to break them down, so the sugar hits the blood stream super-fast, triggering the release of insulin. This gives us a burst of energy, but that instant high is followed by a low, making us feel tired, lethargic, bad-tempered and heavy-headed. So what does the body crave? More sugar, of course, and so the cycle continues, leaving us exhausted and our willpower low. Crucially for us, of course, all that sugar is stored as fat, mainly around the waist, making sugar the worst culprit for putting on excess weight. So if we can regulate this insulin transport system, then the body will stop storing the fat and start to use these fat stores for energy instead.

Take one simple step

The good news is that making a few simple changes can make all the difference to how we process food and can help us to take back control. We can enjoy the carbohydrates we need for energy, without getting the sugar high, simply by eating only complex carbohydrates. These are carbs that take a long time to break down in the body, slowly releasing the sugar into the blood stream and thus not triggering an insulin response. The odd treat of refined white bread and pasta is fine – but as far as our daily diet is concerned, we should stick to the complex carbs. This basic choice is something everyone should adopt in order to achieve better health, and it should always be the first step to take towards achieving your natural, healthy weight and stopping yo-yo dieting and binge eating. If you only make one change to your diet, swapping to complex carbohydrates is the best life-time improvement you can make.

So start right away by not buying them, then you won't be tempted when you see sugary things, cakes, biscuits or refined, sugar-coated cereals in the cupboard. Opt for heavy wholegrain, rye or wholemeal bread … the darker and grainier the better. Stock up on oats and nuts. And, of course, go for fresh vegetables that will give you all the goodness you need.

So now you are all set … let's get started.

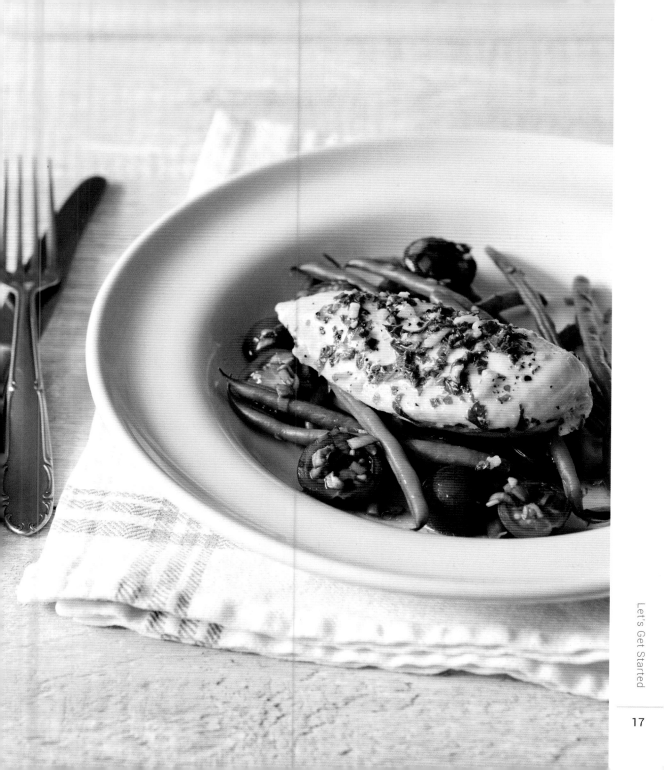

THE FIVE-DAY BODY PREPARATION PLAN

This brings us on to the preparation stage of the plan, which basically sets your body up for the diet itself. I'm going to be honest with you and say that this step is likely to be the hardest part, because it represents the first major step on your journey to a healthier lifestyle and slimmer you, and setting out on something new takes courage.

But just think of the advantages and that will spur you on and give you the energy you need. If you stick to the plan, you can look better, feel better and be healthier than you may have ever been before! That's something worth aiming for. Plus the really good news is that once this step is over, the rest will be easy. You will soon begin to get used to the diet and incorporate it comfortably into your life. And five days is a very short space of time when you consider the long-term benefits.

Check with your doctor

Please consult with your doctor before you start the preparation plan if you have any history of diabetes or any other health condition. If you have already been diagnosed with diabetes, it is crucial that you talk with your doctor before embarking on any kind of diet plan to make sure that it is suitable for your specific condition. If your doctor gives you the go-ahead, make sure you make regular visits to see them while following the plan. You may find that you need a change in your medication and, obviously, the doctor is the one to monitor and advise on this.

Cut out sugar and carbs

The five-day plan is not necessarily designed for weight loss and you shouldn't be focusing on that. Basically it is a process of weaning yourself off the sugar and stabilizing your blood sugar levels so that you can then gain full control of your diet. The goal is to get your body back into balance and off the sugar rollercoaster in order for you to take full control of your diet. Just remember, food doesn't control you, you control food. When your body is in balance and your hormones aren't fighting against your will, this starts to become apparent.

So, for five days, you need to go cold turkey on sugar and carbohydrates. During these five days, you will be eliminating all foods that impact your blood sugar levels – so no carbohydrates, no caffeine, no alcohol, no sauces or condiments and only specific fruits – and you will be drinking nothing but water and herbal tea. You will be on a diet of fish, chicken, turkey, vegetables, salad, eggs and a little red meat. Remember, it's only for five days and you will never go hungry, so don't panic.

Some people will find this a lot harder than others, but you must persist for the full five days in order to get the best results. Once you have completed the five days, then you can begin to adopt your new lifestyle changes with the full diet plan and diet tricks, and start your journey to a thinner, healthier you.

It is possible that some people may experience withdrawal symptoms while on the five-day plan, such as weakness or tiredness, constipation, headaches and irritability. Others may feel bloated and gassy until their digestive system adjusts to the increased fibre intake. These symptoms should only last for three to five days, so stick with it.

In the future, if you feel that your eating is getting out of control again and you're starting to have cravings for junk food, you can rerun the five-day plan. It might also be a good idea to repeat it at the beginning of each year after indulging over the party season.

Foods to eat during the five-day plan

The lists of foods in this section (see page 20) includes everything you are allowed to eat during these five days. You can only eat what is on the list and nothing else, so take a copy to the supermarket with you and get creative in the kitchen. Mix it up to make salads, stews, soups and stir-fries.

Basically, you will be eating a portion of meat or fish with plenty of fresh vegetables to make sure you feel full. That gives you ample scope for variety and interest and there will be no need for you to be hungry while on the plan. You should also drink plenty of water.

Meat, fish and eggs

You can eat eggs and all kinds of meat and fish that are fresh or frozen. That doesn't include pre-packed sandwich meats, sausages, burgers or anything like that – only pure meats and fish with nothing added. Tinned fish is acceptable as long as it is tinned in spring water only.

Do remember, however, not to overdo the meat. Remember that one portion is only the size of your palm; any more is too much.

Vegetables and fruit

For the five-day plan, you can eat plenty of the following vegetables and fruits to fill you up.

- artichokes
- asparagus
- aubergines
- bean sprouts
- bok choi
- broccoli
- brussels sprouts
- cabbage
- cauliflower
- celery

- courgettes
- cucumbers
- green beans
- greens
- leeks
- lemons
- lettuce
- limes
- mangetout
- mushrooms

- okra
- onions
- peppers (red, yellow, orange or green, jalapeño, etc.)
- radishes
- spinach
- tofu
- tomatoes (go easy on these)
- turnips
- yellow squash

Other items allowed

Use these in moderation to add interest to your menus and remember to drink plenty of water.

- apple cider vinegar (for salad dressing) (not balsamic vinegar)
- black pepper
- butter
- fish stock

- flaxseed oil (for salad dressing)
- green tea
- hard cheese (in small quantities)
- herbal teas
- herbs and spices
- lemon juice

- mayonnaise (1 tbsp per day)
- meat stock
- olive oil (for cooking)
- olives
- soured cream
- water

Get ready to implement the diet tricks

Then there's my 10 diet tricks (see pages 22–33), which represent small changes to your lifestyle and eating habits that will make a huge difference to your waistline. They are extra ways to speed up weight loss that are simple to adopt and very effective. Combined with the low-carb principles, they will teach you how to be your natural, trim self and stay slim without fad diets or starve-binge cycles.

Good luck! Stick to the following New Low-Carb Diet plan and you will succeed.

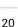

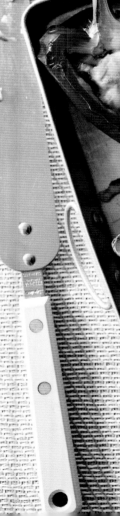

DIET TRICK 1: Maintain Stable Blood Sugar Levels

Once you have completed the five-day plan, you will have weaned yourself off sugar and eliminated cravings. Diet trick 1 is to learn to maintain this new-found blood sugar stability, so that weight loss proceeds naturally, by eliminating the foods that cause the blood sugar levels to increase too quickly. This doesn't have to be difficult. You just need to rethink your food choices and stick to them!

Choose Red for complex carbs

Carry on eating the foods from the five-day plan, but begin to add some complex carbohydrates. While it is important that you don't overdo carbohydrates when trying to lose weight, they do provide you with energy, vitamins and minerals. The best way to ensure that you aren't hindering your weight loss is to have carbohydrates only at breakfast. Using this diet plan in the clinic, we found this was the best way to speed up weight loss while not denying yourself favourite foods – a sure-fire way to send you back to the old ways of eating. So enjoy your carbohydrates at breakfast, making sure that you are choosing the right kind from the Red section of the food lists (see page 39).

As well as changing your food choices, there are also a few additional ways to help you stabilize your blood sugar levels. These simple tricks can also be easily incorporated into your daily life.

Make sure you are getting your oats

The first one is simple: make sure you incorporate oats into your daily diet. Oats are a fantastic source of protein, fibre and the all-important beta glucans, which have been shown in many studies to help stabilize blood sugar levels. So oats should always be your number one choice at breakfast if you want to take full advantage of every trick to speed up your weight loss.

Chromium and the glucose tolerance factor

Chromium is known for its usefulness in stabilizing blood sugar levels as it is thought to enhance the action of insulin in the breakdown of food. If your levels of chromium are already depleted, it is quite difficult to get a high enough dose from natural foods to make up the difference, so you should think about taking some additional GTF chromium as a supplement at this point.

Chromium is a very important nutrient that is known as the 'glucose tolerance factor'. It is thought that as many as one in 10 people could actually be deficient in chromium, which is a huge contributing factor towards weight gain and diabetes. Studies have clearly confirmed that daily supplementation with chromium can lead to significant improvements in body composition in which lean muscle mass increases, resulting in more fat being burnt. Interestingly, these results have been shown to be particularly significant in individuals who haven't even made any specific lifestyle changes, such as dieting or increasing exercise levels – although don't go thinking that you can get out of exercising by popping a chromium supplement instead!

As well as taking a supplement, it is worth adding foods to your diet that contain chromium. The best source is brewer's yeast, which you can find in yeast spreads. If you are one of those who hate them, you can try adding a spoonful to a stew or casserole for some extra flavour and saltiness.

Another useful addition is cinnamon, which has also been shown to have a huge impact on stabilizing blood sugar levels, so try sprinkling it on top of your oats in the morning.

The importance of protein and fibre

Protein is also important in this equation as it has a huge contribution to stabilizing blood sugar levels. Compared to simple sugars and carbohydrates, protein, like fat, takes a lot longer to be broken down in the stomach and therefore leaves us feeling fuller for longer. Protein is also excellent for stabilizing blood sugar levels because it contains no sugar and is digested slowly once eaten, providing us with a good, slow release of energy without the blood sugar rise and insulin release.

We can actually enhance this benefit still further by adding a good amount of fibre with the protein in each meal. This gives bulk in the stomach and so makes you feel fuller, quicker. This combination has the added benefit of preventing constipation, which can sometimes happen on a low-carb, high-protein diet. It is very important, however, that you limit red meat and dairy to just a few times a week. These contain high levels of saturated fat and so should always be the second choice after heart-healthy choices of fish, turkey and chicken.

Diet trick 1
Maintain your blood sugar levels to prevent storage of fat by only eating complex carbohydrates.

DIET TRICK 2: Fat Isn't the Enemy

It sounds logical to target a weight-loss campaign at eliminating fat from the diet, but as the years have passed and we have learned more about the human body, weight loss and weight gain, it is now obvious that this isn't the straightforward answer. There is now an increasing weight of scientific evidence showing that the fat in the food we eat isn't necessarily the real problem.

Although weight for weight, fat has more calories than sugar and any carbohydrate, it is the sugar and carbohydrate that is the bane of all our lives, and is causing a nation of sugar addicts while fuelling the current obesity epidemic. Fat, on the other hand, is exceptionally good at slowing down digestion, while providing us with vitamins A, D, E and K.

Low fat sends you straight on to the yo-yo diet

As a dieter, the most self-destructive thing you can probably do is to buy low-fat, fat-free, light or extra-light diet food products. These foods generally have the fat replaced by sugar (or even worse Aspartame) due to its lower density of calories. So while it does mean that you are then eating fewer calories for the same quantity of food, as those calories are coming in the form of a huge sugar hit, your body will quickly store the excess sugar as fat … then you are back on the now-familiar cycle of blood sugar dip, cravings for another sugar hit, and so on. Willpower and control then go out of the window and you head straight for the junk food, so you put on more weight and buy more diet and fat-free products. This has led me to wonder whether there could be a direct link between these low-fat and fat-free products and the current diabetes epidemic.

Self-serving diet industry

If this is the diet industry's ploy, then it is working very well; if the products you buy to help you lose weight actually help you to maintain your weight, then you are likely to remain on a weight-reducing diet. You buy more products, the cycle continues and they hit the jackpot! So the moral of this story is simple: *if you are going to eat something, eat the original, full-fat version, but just less of it*. If you do this, you will get the benefit of a slower breakdown of the food in the body, so there will be no blood sugar highs and lows and no increased fat stores, but valuable fuel instead.

As an added benefit, you will be consuming something closer to the original product that hasn't been stripped of its essential fat-soluble vitamins, such a vitamin D, in which so many of us are beginning to become deficient.

The best fats to choose

Start by checking the labels, and concentrate on including monounsaturated fats and omega-3 from fish in your diet. Monounsaturated fats are like the 'Supermen' of all fats and are an essential part of a healthy diet. They are needed daily in the body for pretty much all your body's systems to work effectively and can help reverse any damage already done by an excess of saturated fats.

Monounsaturated fats come from foods such as canola oil, corn oil, groundnut oil, olive oil, safflower oil, sesame oil, sunflower oil, popcorn, wholegrain wheat, cereal, oatmeal and avocados. You also find it in nuts and seeds.

Polyunsaturated fats should be eaten regularly in small amounts; they are also found in nuts and seeds as well as fish. Saturated fats should only be eaten in moderation and the sole source should be meat and dairy, which naturally contain some fats. You are already avoiding processed foods, which often contain high levels of saturated fats. Trans fats should be avoided altogether; they are also most commonly found in processed foods.

Symptoms of a deficiency

If you are deficient in essential fats, there are many potential symptoms: high cholesterol, high blood pressure, poor circulation, dry, flaky or cracking skin, other skin conditions, flaky nails, behavioural problems in children, adult acne, poor wound healing, joint pain, dandruff, depression, dry mouth and frequent colds, as well as cravings for fatty foods. If you have any of these symptoms it may be a good idea to take an omega-3 fish oil supplement daily for a while to bring up your levels while introducing some good fats into your diet.

It is very common for long-term dieters to be deficient in many vitamins and minerals as a result of restricting their food intake and following unhealthy diets that are poor in nutrients. If you have any kind of symptom that is unusual or worrying – thinning hair, skin problems, poor memory or mood swings – the chances are that it is due to a deficiency of a nutrient or two. This could actually be holding back your weight loss and so should be remedied as soon as possible.

Diet trick 2
Make sure your body gets enough of the right kind of fats.

DIET TRICK 3: Improve Your Mood & Stop Comfort Eating

I'm sure we've all reached for that bar of chocolate when we've been feeling low, or eaten more than we should because we tend to lose motivation and willpower from time to time. And most of us probably gain a little extra weight during the winter months. This is due to the simple fact that less sunshine means you are producing less of the happy hormone, serotonin, and a decline in serotonin means a decline in mood and motivation.

Boosting the happy hormone

It therefore makes perfect sense to boost your serotonin levels so that you stay happy, motivated and energetic throughout those dark winter months or in those inevitable times in our lives when we are pressured at work or things don't seem to be going quite the way you would like them to.

The good news is that we don't need to move to a sunnier climate – or change our job – to achieve this. The sun isn't the only way that you can increase your serotonin levels; this can also be achieved by our diet and also by supplements.

The amino acid tryptophan is converted to serotonin once in the body, so eating foods rich in tryptophan will increase your serotonin levels naturally. Turkey, fish, chicken, cottage cheese, nuts, cheese, eggs and beans are all good candidates, so be sure to include these in your regular diet throughout the year to keep up your happy hormone levels. And if you do find that you are feeling a little low and lacking in willpower, then head for these foods first.

If you find you are struggling to include a good selection of these foods in your diet, or perhaps you just want a quick and easy fix, then a supplement of 5HTP can be very helpful for a quick boost with fast results.

Finally, and most importantly, you need to be getting out into the fresh air. Try to incorporate at least a 20-minute fast-paced walk every day as this will boost your mood, energy, motivation and more importantly … burn fat!

Diet trick 3
Eat foods rich in nutrients that boost your happy hormone. This will improve your energy levels, boost your willpower and motivation and prevent comfort eating for ever!

DIET TRICK 4: Boost Your Metabolism to Help Burn Fat

As we get older our metabolisms gradually slow down, making us burn calories more slowly and gain weight more easily. By increasing our rate of metabolism, we also increase our basal metabolic rate, which is the amount of energy our bodies use at rest, so we burn more calories when doing nothing. So how can you boost your metabolism so you burn more calories during the day?

- Exercise – find something you enjoy and go for it.
- Eat regularly and don't skip meals … especially breakfast. This ensures that your metabolism is constantly burning at a steady rate.
- Include plenty of protein in your diet to keep you feeling fuller for longer and help with fat burning.
- Do include fibre in your diet. Although it is a type of carbohydrate, fibre takes a long time to digest and so won't impact your blood sugar levels. Plus it prevents constipation, and the added boost in metabolism will result in better circulation so you'll feel warmer during the cold winter months. The best choices are lower-carbohydrate, fibre-rich foods such as nuts, seeds and non-starchy vegetables such as leafy greens, celery, broccoli, cauliflower, tomatoes and peppers.
- Try to drink about 3 litres/105fl oz/12 cups of mineral water during the day. Water helps prevent false hunger pangs, stops your body storing excess water and helps speed up your metabolism.
- Caffeine and green tea can also increase metabolic rate. Drink plenty of green tea, but no more than three coffees or black teas a day. A black coffee before a workout could help you burn more calories.
- Finally, spicy foods have been shown to increase metabolism for hours after you have eaten, so try adding some chilli, cayenne pepper, black pepper, turmeric, ginger or jalapeños to your meals.

Avoiding hypothyroidism

The thyroid gland is vital in regulating metabolism but it needs a good supply of iodine, which can be deficient in a poor diet. The best source is seaweed – I use nori seaweed to replace bread wraps and make sushi – or try a kelp supplement, but check first with your doctor if you are on medication.

Diet trick 4
Eat foods that speed up your metabolism and burn fat quicker for faster weight loss.

DIET TRICK 5: Improve Your Energy Levels & Get Walking

You don't need to sweat it out at the gym to lose weight and maintain it. Although weight training is a great way to build muscle and speed up your metabolism, I understand why most people can't think of anything worse!

But that's okay, because the best way to burn fat is with low-intensity exercise such as a fast-paced walk. A 20–30-minute fast walk every day will really speed up your weight loss and tone your legs and bum. First thing in the morning, before breakfast, is the best time to go and this will then keep your metabolism burning strongly for the rest of the day. If you're not a morning person, then maybe try taking your trainers to work and popping out during your lunch break, or perhaps try parking your car 15 minutes away from work so that you have to walk from there and back every day.

Topping up your B vitamins

You have probably already found that your energy levels have improved drastically since stabilizing your blood sugar levels, but if you still feel a little lethargic and are lacking the energy to exercise, then it could be due to low B vitamin levels. B vitamins are essential for the utilization of energy from food and they can be depleted from the body easily if you are eating a poor diet or are under a lot of stress. The great news is that you will already be getting these from your new diet plan and so your stores will soon be replenished, giving you back lots of energy.

B vitamins are found in turkey, liver, tuna, chilli peppers, lentils, bananas, potatoes and tempeh (soya based). In addition, brewer's yeast, meat, dairy products and eggs are high in vitamin B12, while oats, barley, wheat bran, avocado, salmon, Brazil nuts (and other nuts, too) are also good sources of B vitamins. That gives you plenty of choice and enables you to ring the changes while still making sure you are getting your recommended intake.

If you want a quick morning boost to get you going, you can try supplementing with a B vitamin complex tablet, but always make sure that you take this in the morning with breakfast as taking it at night can keep you awake.

Diet trick 5

Eat foods to boost energy release, and incorporate walking into your daily routine.

DIET TRICK 6: Bring On the Dairy!

Many people are under the impression that you should cut out all dairy products to lose weight. Since they are high in fat and calories, this does sound logical but, in fact, they have been shown to assist in weight loss. It is thought that the calcium binds to fat in the body, making you excrete it rather than absorb it. Natural yogurt is one of the best sources so should be included in your diet every day. A couple of teaspoons on top of most meals works really well.

Diet trick 6
Eat a little natural yogurt daily to help decrease fat absorption from food.

DIET TRICK 7: Fill Up with Calorie-Burning Foods

Certain foods require more energy for the body to break down than they contain, so you can make them part of your everyday meals in large servings, eat them as snacks or cook in soups or stews.

- asparagus
- beetroot
- broccoli
- cabbage
- carrots
- cauliflower
- celery
- chilli peppers (hot)
- cucumbers
- dandelion leaves
- garlic
- green beans
- kale
- lemons
- lettuce
- onions
- radishes
- spinach
- turnips
- watercress

So tuck in and eat as much as you like. You don't need to go hungry with these foods around.

Diet trick 7
Eat as much of these calorie-burning foods as you want to help you feel full.

DIET TRICK 8: No Carbs After Breakfast, No Food After 7pm

There are many no-carb and low-carb diets to choose from, which can be successful in the short term for a number of reasons.

- Cutting out a major food group will significantly reduce your calorie intake.
- You'll eat more protein in its place, which will keep you fuller for longer and prevent cravings.

In practice, however, cutting out carbohydrates completely is unsustainable. Inevitably, you'll go back to eating carbohydrates sooner or later, then you'll put all the weight straight back on. Deprivation is never a good basis on which to maintain your weight throughout life; the key is to allow yourself a little in moderation.

Keep your breakfast carbs

When it comes to the relationship between weight loss and carbohydrates, I strongly believe that the best time to enjoy carbs is at breakfast times, making sure your lunches and evening meals are based on a protein such as fish or meat with lots of salad or vegetables. By structuring your meals in this way, you will automatically reduce your daily calorie intake significantly without having to cut out any food groups or deny yourself something you really enjoy.

Of course, you now understand why you should only choose complex carbs that won't give you a sugar rush, then leave you hungry and craving more.

Seven o'clock curfew

After your dinner in the evening is the worst time that you can eat because the calories won't be burnt off as effectively when you're sitting down and relaxing all evening. By the time you go to bed, you should be just a little bit hungry. Have half a glass of warm milk before you turn in. This will take away any hunger pangs and help you to fall asleep easily while supplying you with slow-release energy throughout the night. If your body doesn't have to worry about digesting food during the night, it can concentrate on its primary job of repairing your body. Plus, you'll be ravenous when you wake up in the morning.

Eating out on a diet

Of course, this diet trick is difficult to follow if you are eating out … but hey, life is too short to make yourself miserable, so allow yourself an evening off every so often for a night out with a little indulgence. If you're a bit of a social bunny and regularly meet friends for dinner, maybe try swapping this for lunchtime catch-ups over the weekend instead. This way you are less tempted by alcohol – and the calories that come with it – and will be more inclined to go for a dish that is a little lighter. Also it is better to have the heaviest meal of the day earlier and a lighter meal in the evening as this gives your body more time to digest the food before bed. If you over-indulge a little at lunch, then you can make up for it by going lighter with your evening meal.

If you are going out for dinner, try to stick to these rules:

- Always resist temptation to nibble at the bread on the table … this is a huge diet no-no. It's far too easy to eat more than you need without even realizing it.
- Skip the starter or share something small and light – and carbohydrate-free.
- Choose a white meat or fish dish, accompanied by either salad or vegetables, with no carbohydrate, so no potatoes, chips, rice, pasta or bread.
- Have a coffee (which is an appetite-suppressant and also a bit of a treat, so is fine in moderation) – or perhaps a green tea if you enjoy it – and a spoonful of someone else's dessert rather than a whole dessert.
- Another option is to share a dessert with someone if it's a special occasion. Just remember: 'A moment on the lips … a life time on the hips!', as my mother used to say. So really think about whether you truly need it before you help yourself.
- Take it easy with the booze as alcohol is extremely high in calories. Again this should be reserved for the occasional treat.

Diet trick 8

Don't eat any carbohydrates after breakfast and stick to a food curfew at 7pm, giving your body time to digest the food you have eaten before you go to sleep.

DIET TRICK 9: Think About Drink!

When it comes to losing weight, many people are so busy thinking about what they can and can't eat that they forget all about what they are drinking. Consuming calories from drinks is unnecessary and can easily be stopped. The worst culprits are fizzy drinks and fruit juices that are packed with sugar and sweeteners.

Fruit juice and fizzy drinks

Although fruit juices can be a great source of vitamins and minerals, I'd advise that you avoid these all together. Just having three glasses a day can equate to 450g/1lb a week in weight gain and, in fact, many people who drink fresh juices and fizzy drinks could lose weight just by cutting these out of their diet, even if they make no other changes.

Fizzy drinks are completely unnecessary. Even the sugar-free varieties with lots of sweeteners play havoc with your blood sugar levels, while large quantities of added sweeteners and caffeine will later lead to cravings when you have the sugar/caffeine come-down. Again these should be saved for the occasional glass and should by no means be for everyday drinking.

So what are the better options?

Make sure you're drinking enough fluid in the form of water and herbal teas. This will prevent your body from holding water (fluid retention), prevent false hunger pangs, keep your metabolism burning in between meals, give you a fresher complexion and make you feel great! Be sure to drink about 3 litres/105fl oz/12 cups per day, adding an extra glass for every coffee you have.

Obviously, the first choice would always be mineral water, but if you want to add a little flavour to it, you could try a squeeze of lemon or lime.

Another great choice is herbal teas. These can be brewed, then cooled and watered down a little to make a cold drink. A good choice is a weight-loss herbal tea mix, which you can get from health food shops. These often have gentle diuretic effects, which will help rid you of excess water retention, thus improving any feelings of bloating and also shedding some water weight. But don't overdo it with these, as they could leave you depleted in vitamins.

Diet trick 9

No more fruit juices or fizzy drinks! Drink at least 3 litres/105fl oz/12 cups water or herbal tea a day.

DIET TRICK 10: Don't Be Greedy

When it comes to changing your eating habits, a big thing that you have to re-evaluate is portion size. We all know how easy it is to go for seconds and carry on eating until we can't possibly fit in another morsel, but this really has to stop! As a child you were probably encouraged to finish up everything on your plate and then given the reward of dessert if the plate was emptied. Things like this have conditioned us into believing that we have to eat a huge amount of food to be full, when really our stomachs are only the size of our fists! So every time we eat until we are uncomfortably full we are stretching our stomachs to their limits. And, like a balloon, once stretched over and over again, it begins to keep this new shape. It then takes more food in order to fill it … and so our portions get bigger and bigger, since it now takes more food in order to feel satisfied.

This habit needs to be broken and you'll have to train yourself to do it. It's not easy, but once you get the hang of it, it'll soon become second nature.

The best way to control portion size is to stick to the following guidelines: a palm-size piece of meat and a tablespoon of oil or sauce.

You also need to remember to eat as slowly as possible and focus on what you are eating. Don't sit in front of the TV or the food will be gone without you even noticing. Sit somewhere quiet and enjoy your meal, chew properly and savour every mouthful.

Be mindful as you are eating, really focus on the moment and on your meal and enjoy the experience. Try to think about how hungry you are before you start and then acknowledge the feeling when you are full. When you feel comfortably full, then take your plate away immediately and dispose of any food remaining so that it can't tempt you again. It's all about listening to your stomach and not your mouth, with no distractions around you.

By learning this control, you'll then be able to enjoy things like chocolate in small quantities and have the willpower to stop when you have had enough. It's great to be able to allow yourself some chocolate every so often – good-quality dark chocolate, made with at least 70 per cent cocoa solids, makes a delicious treat, and is lower in sugar and saturated fat than milk chocolate as well as richer in antioxidants. Slowly savour about four squares – that is enough – then stop. Your willpower will need to kick in but you'll soon get the hang of it.

Diet trick 10
Eat small portions slowly and regularly and never go back for seconds.

THE CANDIDA FACTOR

If you have followed the diet plan for a few weeks but are not losing weight, it is possible that this is due to a candida overgrowth in the body. Candida is a yeast that can easily thrive anywhere that is warm and moist, with a bit of sugar or alcohol, so the chances are that if you have been eating a high-carb diet or drinking alcohol, then your body will be like a breeding ground for candida to multiply and thrive.

For many people, the first signs of a yeast problem may be a yeast infection, such as athlete's foot, nail infections, thrush or a flaky skin rash; or it may be headaches, irritability, heartburn or flatulence. But if you are thinking that you have never had any visible candida infections so you don't have to worry, then you could be wrong! Less sweating or a more effective cleaning routine to prevent prolonged warm, damp conditions on the skin may mean there are no external symptoms, but it certainly doesn't mean candida isn't hiding somewhere internally, where it can cause damage if left for a prolonged time.

When overgrown in the gut, candida spores damage the intestinal wall and over time this damage can lead to a condition called leaky gut. As the name suggests, food particles, toxins and allergens can leak out of the gut into the blood stream. Your gut is there as a barrier to prevent this and to support your immune system in the fight against viruses and bacteria entering the body. When the gut is leaky, it lets in harmful allergens that would usually pass through without a reaction. This, in turn, can gradually lead to new allergies to foods that were once enjoyed. As well as the health problems that can be caused by this overgrowth, it can also play havoc with your weight.

What to do

In order to starve the candida:

- Avoid all yeast products, such as yeast spreads, beef spread, vinegars, mushrooms, processed meats and processed fish.
- Avoid cheeses, butter, eggs, mayonnaise, soured cream and soy sauce.
- Take a course of probiotic supplements. This will fine-tune your digestive system and recolonize it with good bacteria, giving you a fast boost.
- Increase your intake of asparagus, garlic, leek, onion and artichoke to allow the type of fibre they contain to work as a prebiotic to restore the balance.

THE NEW LOW-CARB FOOD PLAN

Now that you have completed the preparation plan, you should already be feeling mentally stronger, more positive and in control. You'll also have read the diet tricks and be ready to put them into practice. By using my recipes and following this colour-coded plan, you can educate yourself and your body to make the right food choices that will transform your attitudes towards food.

You will see quick results, but this is so much more than a quick-fix diet. It is a set of guidelines for a new approach to achieving optimal nutrition and health for life. If you stick to this plan for about three months, you will understand where you were making wrong choices before. You will need scales to weigh foods until you get used to portion quantities but you'll soon be able to judge your meals without them. The idea is not to focus on weighing and counting but to work towards a point where you naturally follow a healthy diet because you understand what good eating is about.

All the recipes in this book fit into this plan. You can use them until you feel confident enough to start creating your own meals. Some recipes give you a bonus – an extra spoonful of yogurt or a slightly larger quantity of something – so that the dishes are as delicious as they are healthy. Such variations are part of normal healthy eating and will even out over the course of a few days.

Meal plans

Select from the pre-calculated recipes or create your own meals by picking the designated number of food items from the colour-coded groups. Everyone uses the same plan, but men can have an afternoon shake. Plus you can have as much from the free foods list as you like.

Breakfast
Half a **Blue** plus one **Yellow** plus one **Red** (such as 1 slice of ham, 1 tablespoon of butter, 4 oat cakes)
Lunch
One **Blue** plus one **Yellow** plus one **Green**
Afternoon shake (for men only) 1 tablespoon of whey protein isolate powder mixed with a little water and 100ml/3½fl oz/scant ½ cup natural yogurt
Dinner
One **Blue** plus two **Yellow** plus one **Green**
Nightcap
Half a mug of warm milk

THE FOOD GROUPS

Here are the lists of foods by colour category: purple for the free foods, blue for protein, yellow for fats, red for carbs and green for vegetables. Download the lists from www.thenewlowcarbdiet.com, print them out and stick them on the fridge door for easy reference. Once a week, you can treat yourself to a dessert from my recipes, which are formulated not to impact your blood sugar levels.

Free foods

This should become your favourite section since you can basically use these foods wherever you like and add them to any meal. Where the daily maximum quantity is important, that is included.

Flavourings and other foods
- 2 anchovy fillets
- balsamic vinegar
- black pepper
- brewer's yeast spread
- capers
- coffee
- 1 tsp cornflour
- 1 egg white
- fish sauce
- gravy granules
- herbal teas
- herbs and spices
- lemon or lime juice
- low-calorie cooking oil spray
- a dash of semi-skimmed milk
- mint sauce
- miso soup
- mustard
- nori seaweed
- 5 olives

- 1 tbsp oyster sauce
- 1 tbsp passata
- pickled gherkins, onions and cabbage
- 1 tbsp salsa
- shirataki noodles
- soy sauce (reduced salt)
- stock or stock cubes
- 2 sun-dried tomatoes
- tabasco sauce
- tea
- 200g/7oz tinned tomatoes
- 1 tsp tomato purée
- wine or rice vinegar
- Worcestershire sauce
- 2 tsp natural yogurt

Vegetables
- asparagus
- bean sprouts
- beetroot

- broccoli
- cabbage
- carrots
- cauliflower
- celeriac
- celery
- chilli peppers
- cucumbers
- garlic
- green beans
- kale
- lettuce (all varieties)
- onions
- radishes
- rocket
- spinach
- spring onions
- stevia powder
- tomatoes
- turnips
- watercress

Blue – protein

This is the protein section, which should form the centre of your meals. Mix these up and combine them in imaginative ways.

Cheese

- 50g/1¾oz blue cheese
- 60g/2¼oz Brie
- 60g/2¼oz Camembert
- 50g/1¾oz Cheddar cheese
- 200g/7oz cottage cheese
- 50g/1¾oz cream cheese
- 80g/2¾oz feta cheese
- 60g/2¼oz mozzarella cheese
- 40g/1½oz Parmesan cheese
- 80g/2¾oz soft goats' cheese

Dairy and vegetarian

- 2 eggs
- 3 vegetarian sausages (good quality)
- 200g/7oz firm tofu
- 50g/1¾oz (2 scoops) whey protein isolate powder (a dietary supplement made from milk powder)

Fish

- 100g/3½oz oily fish, including mackerel and herring
- 150g/5½oz rainbow trout
- 130g/4½oz salmon
- 160g/5½oz sardines
- 200g/7oz seafood, including crab, prawns and squid
- 100g/3½oz smoked salmon
- 150g/5½oz swordfish
- 150g/5½oz tinned tuna in spring water
- 200g/7oz tuna steak
- 200g/7oz white fish, including cod, haddock, hake, plaice and pollack

Meat and poultry

- 4 slices of bacon
- 100g/3½oz lean beef or minced beef
- 180g/6¼oz chicken breast
- 4 slices of cooked or prepacked chicken or turkey
- 150g/5½oz duck
- 2 slices of ham
- 150g/5½oz lamb fillet
- 10 thin slices of Parma ham or other cured ham
- 70g/2½oz pork
- 70g/2½oz minced pork
- 200g/7oz turkey
- 150g/5½oz minced turkey
- 100g/3½oz lean steak
- 130g/4½oz venison

Nuts and seeds

- 35g/1¼oz/scant ¼ cup almond flour
- 35g/1¼oz/scant ¼ cup nuts, including almonds, raw unsalted peanuts, cashew nuts, pistachio nuts
- 2 tbsp peanut butter (no added sugar) or nutella
- 40g/1½oz/¼ cup sesame seeds
- 35g/1¼oz/heaped ¼ cup sunflower seeds
- 30g/1oz/scant ¼ cup walnuts

Yellow – fats

These foods are rich in fat – good and bad. You need some fat in your diet but try to choose monounsaturated and polyunsaturated fats, and have the unhealthy saturated fats only occasionally (see pages 24–25). If you prefer to weigh the nuts, you are allowed 15–20g/½–¾oz, which is 100kcals.

Cheese and dairy
- 25g/1oz blue cheese
- 1 tbsp butter
- 30g/1oz Brie
- 30g/1oz Camembert
- 20g/¾oz Cheddar cheese
- 100g/3½oz cottage cheese
- 1 heaped tbsp cream cheese
- 2 tbsp crème fraîche
- 2 tbsp double cream
- 40g/1½oz feta cheese
- 40g/1½oz soft goats' cheese
- 200ml/7fl oz/scant 1 cup milk, oat milk, soy milk
- 35g/1¼oz mozzarella cheese
- 20g/¾oz Parmesan cheese
- 3 tbsp soured cream

Meat
- 4 slices of bacon
- 3 slices of Parma ham

Nuts and seeds
- 2 tbsp almonds
- 2 tbsp Brazil nuts
- 2 tbsp cashew nuts
- 2 tbsp flaxseeds
- 2 tbsp hazel nuts
- 2 tbsp macadamia nuts
- 2 tbsp raw unsalted peanuts
- 2 tbsp pine nuts
- 2 tbsp pistachio nuts
- 2 tbsp sesame seeds
- 2 tbsp sunflower seeds
- 2 tbsp walnuts

Sauces, condiments and other foods
- ¼ avocado
- 3 tbsp coconut milk
- 2 tbsp hollandaise sauce
- 2 tbsp horseradish sauce
- 1 tbsp mayonnaise
- 1 tbsp oil, including corn oil, groundnut oil, olive oil, peanut oil, rapeseed oil, sesame oil, sunflower oil
- 100g/3½oz/¾ cup olives
- 1 tbsp peanut butter (no added sugar)
- 1 tbsp pesto
- 1 tbsp tahini
- 3 tbsp white sauce

Who needs additives?

It's actually quite easy to see which foods are not filled with these sneaky little additives that have crept into so many of our foods as colourings, preservatives, flavours and flavour enhancers, sweeteners, texture agents and processing agents. Just glance at the ingredients list on any foods you buy. The longer the list, the more likely the food contains loads of additives that you simply don't need. Put it back and go for the ones with the short list! And if you want to check them out, go to www.thenewlowcarbdiet.com where you will find all the details.

Red – carbohydrates

These are your choices for your breakfast fix of carbohydrate.

Fruit

- 2 apples
- 5 apricots
- 1 banana
- 20 cherries
- 1 grapefruit
- 2 kiwi fruit
- 2 oranges
- 2 peaches
- 2 pears
- 3 plums
- 20 strawberries

Grains

- 2 medium slices of bread, including brown, buckwheat, multigrain, oat, pumpernickel, rye, spelt, stoneground, sourdough, wholewheat
- 4 oat cakes
- 50g/1¾oz/½ cup rolled oats
- 1 wholewheat pitta bread
- 50g/1¾oz/¼ cup brown rice
- 70g/2½oz Shredded Wheat

Green – vegetables

Eat generously of this vegetable section. One serving is up to 4 cups and can be mixed. Remember, of course, that many vegetables appear in the free foods section, giving you a huge variety of vegetables to include in your diet.

Vegetables and fruit

- artichokes
- aubergine
- bok choi
- brussels sprouts
- courgettes
- greens
- leeks
- lemons
- limes
- mangetout
- mushrooms
- okra
- peas (1 cup only once a week)
- peppers (sweet)
- peppers (hot, such as jalapeño, etc.)
- swede (1 cup only once a week)
- sweetcorn (1 cup only once a week)
- yellow squash

Remember, at the end of the day, it comes down to basic science of the human body. If you eat fewer calories than your body needs to function, then you will lose weight. Every human's metabolism works in this same way, so if you really want to, you will lose weight on this diet plan. Always bear in mind that you control what food you eat. Food doesn't control you. Good luck.

CHAPTER 2
BREAKFAST RECIPES

As we all keep hearing, breakfast is the most important meal of the day and this is particularly true if you are trying to lose weight. If we start the day on the right track and eat a good breakfast made up of a complex carbohydrate along with good sources of fat and protein, we then create a slow, steady release of sugar into our system and we avoid any dips in our blood sugar levels before lunch. This means that we can focus on our life and not on our stomachs. All these breakfasts – like these Crunchy Granola Yogurt Pots (see page 46) – are prepared with a balance of complex carbohydrate, protein and fat to ensure the best possible start to the day. Plus the added boost to your metabolism will make doubly sure you don't get any mid-morning hunger pangs to throw you off the diet plan.

Breakfast is the only time of the day when we can incorporate a good source of carbohydrate while on this plan, so make the most of the opportunity. Wake up a little earlier and make the time to take full advantage and enjoy every delicious mouthful.

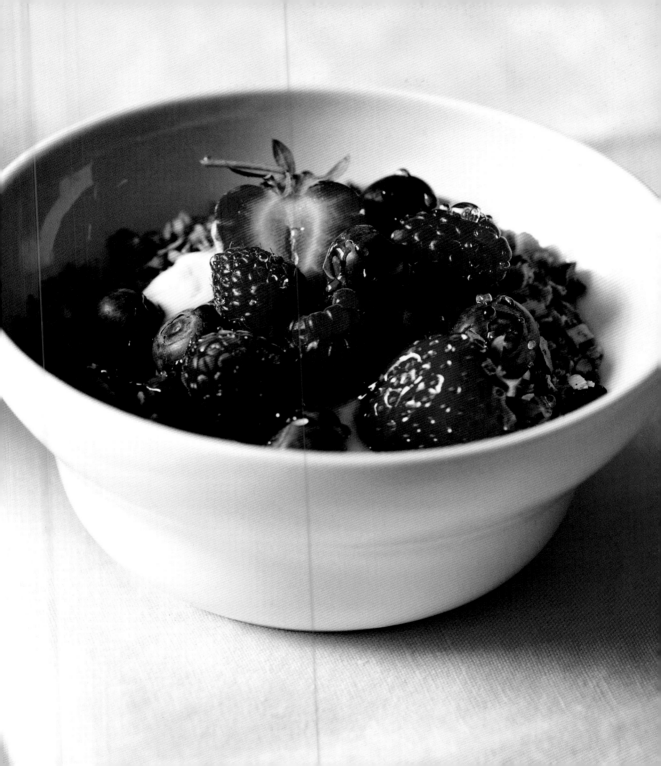

2 apples, peeled, cored and
    quartered
2 pears, peeled, cored and quartered
½ avocado, peeled and pitted

20g/¾oz/scant ¼ cup ground
    almonds
1½ tbsp natural yogurt
2 tsp agave nectar

1 tsp almond extract
1 handful of ice

Fruit & Almond Avocado Smoothie

Serves: 2

Preparation time:
10 minutes

Although this recipe may sound a little unusual, please do give it a try as I know you will be pleasantly surprised!

1　Put all the ingredients into a blender or food processor and blend together until thick and creamy.

2　Pour the smoothie into two large glasses to serve.

2 bananas
200g/7oz strawberries, hulled
400ml14fl oz/scant 1⅔ cups oat milk
1½ tbsp natural yogurt

2 tsp agave nectar
½ tsp ground cinnamon
4 tbsp vanilla whey protein isolate
    powder

Banana & Strawberry Smoothie

Serves: 2

Preparation time:
10 minutes

If you like to have your breakfast on the go, this is a great recipe idea for you. Just blend together the ingredients, then pop the smoothie into a large flask so you can enjoy it on the train or bus on your way to work.

1　Put all the ingredients into a blender or food processor and blend together until thick and creamy.

2　Pour the smoothie into two large glasses to serve.

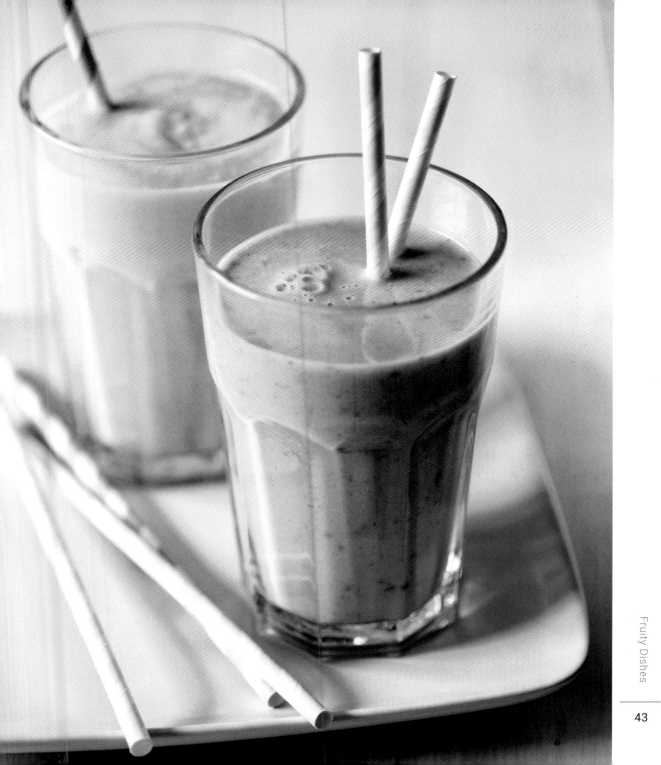

2 red eating apples, peeled, cored
and diced
4 apricots, pitted and diced
1 celery stick, diced

30g/1oz/scant ¼ cup walnuts,
chopped
300ml/10½floz/scant 1¼ cups
natural yogurt

2 tsp lemon juice
2 tsp agave nectar
½ tsp ground cinnamon

Tangy Lemon Yogurt Fruit Salad >

Serves: 2

Preparation time:
10 minutes

This is a great summer recipe, which I think is best enjoyed in the sunshine. It is fresh and light and will fill you up without feeling too heavy. And perhaps it will even bring some sunshine to a rainy morning. Use your favourite red eating apples – something nice and crunchy.

1 Put the apples, apricots, celery and walnuts in a large bowl. Add the yogurt, lemon juice and agave nectar and mix together well.
2 Serve sprinkled with cinnamon.

300g/10½oz blueberries
400g/14oz strawberries, hulled
and diced
1 grapefruit, peeled and diced

1 celery stick, finely chopped
100g/3½oz/1¼ cups desiccated
coconut
2 tsp agave nectar

200ml/7fl oz/scant 1 cup natural
Greek yogurt
½ tsp ground cinnamon

Berries & Citrus with Coconut Yogurt

Serves: 2

Preparation time:
10 minutes

The addition of the coconut makes this into a delicious, exotic cocktail of fresh fruits to set you up for the day.

1 Put the blueberries, strawberries, grapefruit and celery in a large bowl. Stir the coconut and agave nectar into the yogurt and mix together well.
2 Serve the fruit salad topped with the yogurt and finished off with a light sprinkling of cinnamon.

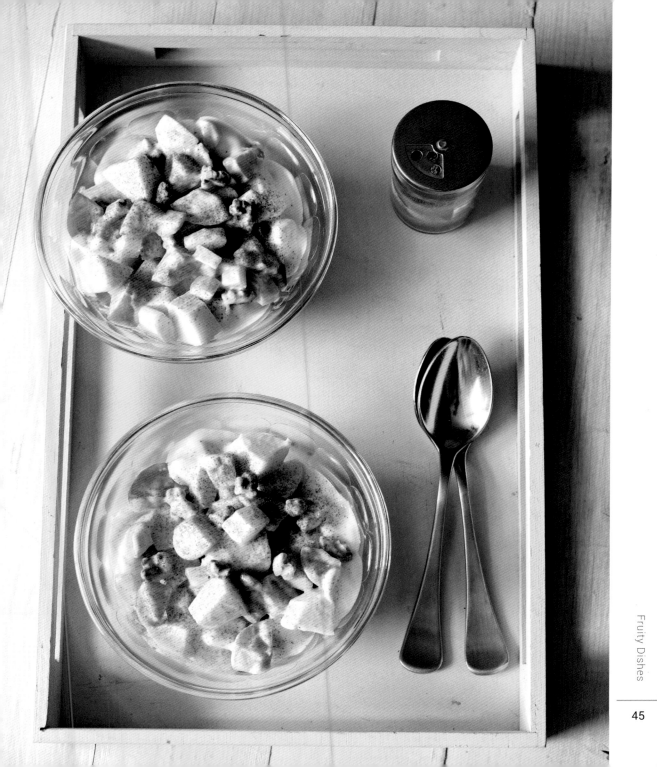

100g/3½oz/1 cup rolled oats

35g/1¼oz/scant ¼ cup almonds, chopped

2 tbsp butter

2 tsp stevia powder

1 tsp vanilla extract

1 tsp ground cinnamon

1½ tbsp natural yogurt

1 tsp agave nectar

2 handfuls of mixed berries, to serve

Crunchy Berry Granola Yogurt Pots

Serves: 2

Preparation time:
10 minutes

Cooking time:
20 minutes

This recipe will be popular with the whole family, with its lovely texture combination of crunchy granola and creamy sweet yogurt. It also uses stevia powder, which is a natural sweetener that you can buy in health food stores. Prepare the granola in advance for a quick-fix nutritious breakfast before work. You can see how good this dish looks on pages 40–41.

1   Preheat the oven to 170°C/325°F/gas 3 and line a baking tray with baking paper. Mix together the oats and chopped almonds in a bowl.

2   Put the butter, stevia powder, vanilla extract and cinnamon in a non-stick saucepan over a low heat and stir until melted and thoroughly combined. Pour over the almond mixture and stir to coat all the dry ingredients. Pour the granola mixture on to the prepared baking tray and spread evenly.

3   Bake for about 10 minutes, then remove the granola from the oven, stir well, then return it to the oven for a further 10 minutes until golden. Leave to cool, then store in an airtight container.

4   Top the yogurt with the granola and a drizzle of agave nectar, then spoon the berries on the top.

NUTRITION NOTES
PER SERVING
• • • • • • • • • • • • • • • • • •
• Calories: 451kcals
• Fat: 27g
• Carbohydrates: 38g

100g/3½oz/1 cup rolled oats

400ml/14fl oz/scant 1⅔ cups oat milk

40g/1½oz/¼ cup almonds

1 tsp ground cinnamon

1 tsp freshly grated nutmeg

½ tsp ground ginger

2 cloves

½ tsp vanilla extract

2 tsp agave nectar

1½ tbsp natural yogurt, to serve

Spiced Almond Porridge

Serves: 2

Preparation time:
5 minutes

Cooking time:
30 minutes

This recipe is an Indian-inspired porridge that is perfect for a cold winter's day. The spices really get your circulation going to keep you feeling warm all morning. Plus, of course, oats make the perfect basis for a slow release of energy so you don't flag by coffee time and resort to a sugar-rush snack.

1   Put all the ingredients except the yogurt in a non-stick saucepan over a low heat and cook for about 30 minutes, stirring regularly, until thick and creamy.

2   Serve topped with a dollop of natural yogurt.

NUTRITION NOTES
PER SERVING

- Calories: 435kcals
- Fat: 18g
- Carbohydrates: 54g

FOR THE ALMOND RYE BREAD

low-calorie cooking oil spray

210ml/7½fl oz/scant 1 cup
lukewarm semi-skimmed milk

1½ tsp dried yeast

2 tbsp stevia powder

250g/9oz/2½ cups rye flour

250g/9oz/2 cups strong white flour,
plus extra for dusting

1 tsp fine sea salt

1 tsp ground cinnamon

25g/1oz/¼ cup ground almonds

FOR THE FRENCH TOAST

1 tbsp butter

½ tsp vanilla extract

½ tsp ground cinnamon

2 eggs, lightly beaten

1 tsp agave nectar

Almond Rye Bread French Toast

Serves: 2

FOR THE BREAD:
Preparation time:
25 minutes, plus
3½ hours rising

Cooking time:
45 minutes

FOR THE FRENCH
TOAST:
Preparation time:
5 minutes

Cooking time:
5 minutes

This classic breakfast recipe is a perfect way to start the day if you like something sweet. If you make it in a breadmaker, put the liquid ingredients, then the dry ingredients in the pan, replacing the yeast with the fast-action variety, and switch on. The loaf cuts into 10 slices so use one slice per serving for your French toast and keep the rest for other breakfasts.

1 To make the bread, grease a large bowl with low-calorie oil spray and line a baking sheet with baking paper. Heat the milk and 175ml/6fl oz/¾ cup of warm water in a saucepan over a low heat. Add the yeast and leave for 10 minutes until frothy.

2 Put the remaining bread ingredients in a mixing bowl and stir until combined. Pour in the yeast mixture and stir well to form a dough. Turn out on to a lightly floured work surface and knead for about 10 minutes, or until the dough is smooth and elastic. Transfer the kneaded dough to the prepared bowl, cover with cling film and a kitchen towel and leave to rise in a warm place for 2½ hours until doubled in size.

3 Knock the air out of the dough, turn it out on to a lightly floured work surface and knead again for 1–2 minutes. Shape the dough into a tight round ball and put it on the prepared baking sheet. Dust the top of the dough with a little flour, cover with a clean kitchen towel and leave to rise in a warm place for a further 45 minutes.

4 Preheat the oven to 180°C/350°F/gas 4. Uncover the bread and bake for 40 minutes until golden brown. Transfer to a wire rack and leave to cool for at least 30 minutes.

5 To make the French toast, cut 2 slices of the bread. Melt the butter in a non-stick frying pan. Beat the vanilla and cinnamon into the eggs in a shallow bowl, then turn the bread slices in the egg so they absorb the liquid. Fry them in the butter for 2 minutes on each side until golden, then serve drizzled with the agave nectar.

NUTRITION NOTES
PER SERVING
••••••••••••••••••

• Calories: 300kcals
• Fat: 14g
• Carbohydrates: 34g

PER BREAD SLICE
••••••••••••••••••

• Calories: 176kcals
• Fat: 3g
• Carbohydrates: 31g

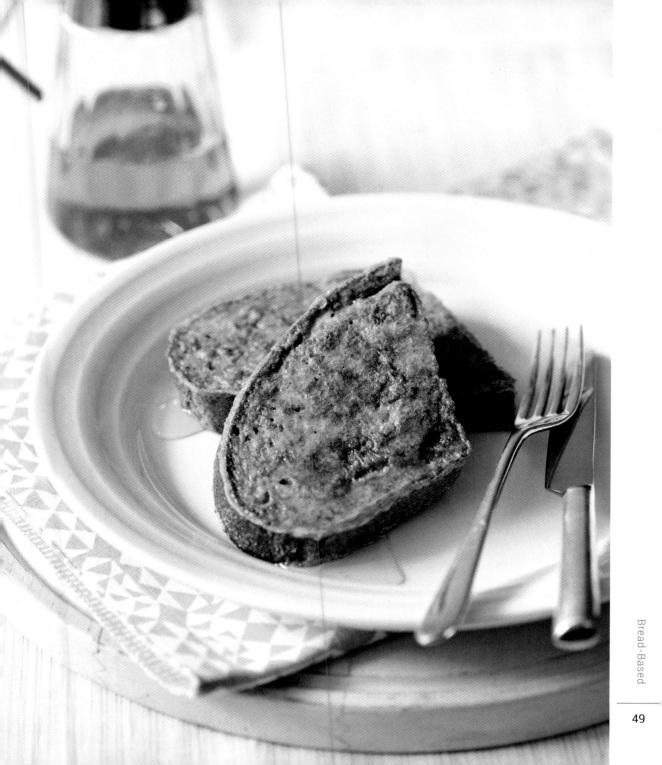

4 medium-thick slices of bacon

2 slices of Olive Soda Bread
  (see page 52)

1 tbsp cream cheese

4 cherry tomatoes, finely chopped

2 chive stalks, finely chopped

freshly ground black pepper

Crispy Bacon & Cream Cheese on Olive Soda Bread

Serves: 2

Preparation time:
5 minutes, plus
making the bread

Cooking time:
15 minutes

This is one of my favourite weekend treats. It's not an everyday breakfast, as we all know bacon isn't the healthiest of options, but once in a while, as part of your overall healthy diet, it is perfectly fine.

1 Preheat the oven to 200°C/400°F/gas 6 and line a baking tray with kitchen foil. Put the bacon on the foil and bake for about 15 minutes, or until crispy.

2 Meanwhile, preheat the grill to high, then toast the bread on both sides.

3 Put the cream cheese in a bowl and stir to soften it slightly, then add the tomatoes and chives and season to taste with pepper. Gently mix all the ingredients together well. Top the hot toast with the cream cheese mixture and finish with the slices of crispy bacon to serve.

NUTRITION NOTES
PER SERVING
·················

• Calories: 238kcals
• Fat: 15g
• Carbohydrates: 13g

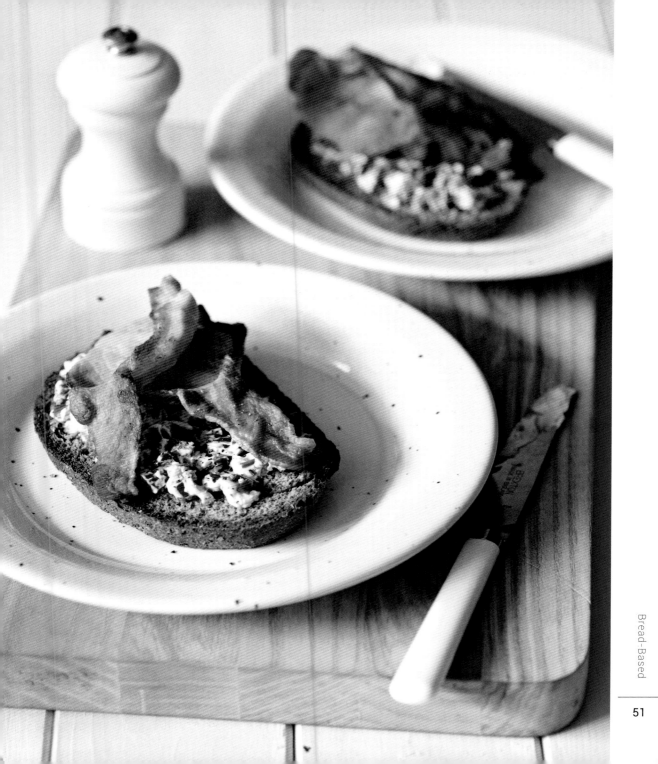

FOR THE OLIVE SODA BREAD

low-calorie cooking oil spray

420g/15oz/scant 3 cups strong
   wholemeal flour, plus extra
   for dusting

1½ tsp baking powder

½ tsp bicarbonate of soda

1 tsp ground cinnamon

4 tbsp butter, cut into small pieces,
   plus extra for greasing

1 small egg, lightly beaten

300ml/10½fl oz/scant 1¼ cups
   natural yogurt

½ tbsp agave nectar

15 pitted black or green olives,
   thinly sliced

FOR THE SCRAMBLED EGG

2 eggs

1 egg white

1 tbsp milk

a pinch of black pepper

50g/1¾oz chorizo, diced

½ red pepper, finely chopped

4 coriander leaves, finely chopped

2 large tomatoes, sliced

Chorizo & Egg on Olive Soda Bread

Serves: 2

FOR THE BREAD:
Preparation time:
15 minutes, plus
3 hours rising

Cooking time:
35 minutes

FOR THE
SCRAMBLED EGG:
Preparation time:
8 minutes

Cooking time:
15 minutes

NUTRITION NOTES
PER SERVING
· · · · · · · · · · · · · · · · · · ·
· Calories: 322kcals
· Fat: 18g
· Carbohydrates: 24g

PER BREAD SLICE
· · · · · · · · · · · · · · · · · · ·
· Calories: 124kcals
· Fat: 7g
· Carbohydrates: 11g

This delicious loaf also works well in your breadmaker. It cuts into 10 slices so use one slice per serving for this Spanish-inspired treat and you'll have plenty for other recipes. This is also a great way to use up slightly stale bread.

1   To make the bread, grease a large bowl with low-calorie oil spray. Mix the flour, baking powder, bicarbonate of soda and cinnamon in a second large bowl. Rub in the butter with your fingertips until the mixture resembles breadcrumbs.

2   Add the remaining bread ingredients and mix to a dough, then transfer to a lightly floured work surface and knead for a few minutes until soft, pliable and no longer sticky. Transfer to the prepared bowl, cover with cling film and a kitchen towel and leave to stand in a warm place for about 3 hours until doubled in size.

3   Preheat the oven to 190°C/375°F/gas 5 and grease a baking sheet. Shape the dough and put on the prepared sheet. Bake for 35 minutes until golden and hollow-sounding when tapped on the base. Cool on a wire rack.

4   Whisk the eggs, egg white, milk and black pepper. Put the chorizo and red pepper in a non-stick saucepan over a low heat and dry-fry for 5 minutes. Add the egg mix and stir continuously for 5 minutes until cooked through, then remove from the heat and stir in the coriander. Transfer the scrambled egg to a serving plate, cover and keep warm. Preheat the grill to high. Add the sliced tomato to the pan and cook for a few minutes on each side until browned. Toast 2 slices of the bread. Top the toast with the scrambled egg and serve with the tomatoes.

100g/3½oz skinless salmon fillet

2 slices of lemon

2 large handfuls of spinach leaves,
   stems removed

2 slices of Wholemeal Walnut Bread
   (see page 59)

2 tbsp olive oil

½ tbsp lemon juice

½ garlic clove

freshly ground black pepper

Lemon Salmon on Walnut Bread

Serves: 2

Preparation time:
10 minutes, plus
making the bread

Cooking time:
25 minutes

Salmon and walnuts are some of the best beauty foods around and if eaten regularly you will really start to notice your skin quality improve. This is just one reason why oily fish should always be your first choice when it comes to meals.

1   Preheat the oven to 180°C/350°F/gas 4. Put a 35cm/14in square of kitchen foil on to a baking tray and put the salmon fillet in the centre. Sprinkle with a twist of pepper and put the lemon slices on top. Wrap the foil loosely around the salmon, rolling and sealing the edges to form an airtight parcel. Bake for about 25 minutes. Unwrap carefully to make sure the salmon is perfectly tender; it should flake easily when tested with a fork.

2   Towards the end of the cooking time, put the spinach in a saucepan with 1 tablespoon of water and cook over a low heat for about 1 minute until just wilted. Drain the spinach well in a sieve or colander, then press down on the spinach with the back of a wooden spoon to remove as much water as possible. Preheat the grill to high and toast the bread on both sides.

3   To make the dressing, put the olive oil, lemon juice and garlic in a small bowl and season with a twist of pepper, then whisk together until thoroughly blended.

4   Divide the spinach between the pieces of toast. Roughly flake the salmon fillet and spread over the top, then drizzle with the olive oil dressing to serve.

NUTRITION NOTES
PER SERVING
• • • • • • • • • • • • • • • • • •
• Calories: 428kcals
• Fat: 23g
• Carbohydrates: 38g

2 large tomatoes, halved

2 tbsp balsamic vinegar

½ avocado, peeled and pitted

a pinch of cayenne pepper

2 slices of Olive Soda Bread
    (see page 52)

160g/5¾oz tinned tuna in spring
    water, drained and flaked

1 handful of rocket leaves

freshly ground black pepper

green tea, to serve (optional)

Tuna Avocado on Olive Soda Bread with Balsamic Roasted Tomatoes

Serves: 2

Preparation time:
10 minutes, plus
making the bread

Cooking time:
20 minutes

This always-perfect combination of tuna and avocado works fantastically with the alkaline taste of the bread against the acidic tang of the tomatoes … a delicious combination that makes a great start to the day. This loaf was made with black olives but you could use green if you prefer.

1 Preheat the oven to 180°C/350°F/gas 4. Put the tomatoes, cut-side up, on a baking tray and sprinkle over half the balsamic vinegar. Roast for 15–20 minutes.

2 Meanwhile, put the avocado and cayenne in a bowl, season to taste with pepper and mash together.

3 When the tomatoes are almost ready, preheat the grill to high, then toast the bread on both sides. Spread evenly with the avocado, then spoon over the tuna. Top with a little rocket, arrange the roasted tomatoes on the side and drizzle with the remaining balsamic vinegar. Serve with green tea, if you like.

NUTRITION NOTES
PER SERVING
• • • • • • • • • • • • • • • •
• Calories: 291kcals
• Fat: 14g
• Carbohydrates: 24g

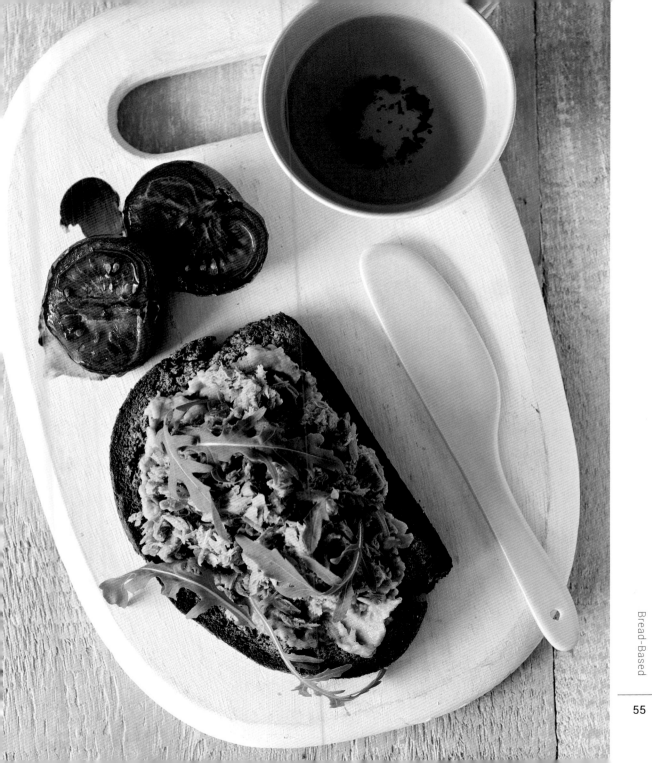

2 eggs

2 slices of Almond Rye Bread
   (see page 48)

2 large handfuls of spinach leaves,
   stems removed

salt and freshly ground black pepper

FOR THE HOLLANDAISE SAUCE

1 tsp apple cider vinegar

a large pinch of white pepper

2 egg yolks

1 tbsp butter

1 tsp lemon juice

Egg & Spinach on Almond Rye Bread with Hollandaise Sauce

Serves: 2

Preparation time:
10 minutes, plus
making the bread

Cooking time:
5 minutes

If you have a little time in the morning, this is a really delicious option. You can make a few servings of the hollandaise at the weekend and use it up over the following few days.

1   To make the hollandaise sauce, put all the sauce ingredients in a small non-stick saucepan over a very low heat and stir continuously for about 5 minutes until the butter has melted and the ingredients have combined to form a thick sauce.

2   Meanwhile, bring a wide, shallow saucepan of lightly salted water to the boil over a high heat, then turn down the heat to low and stir the water vigorously. Break 1 egg into a cup, then slip it into the water. Repeat with the other egg. Simmer for 3–4 minutes until the whites have set but the yolks remain runny.

3   While the eggs are cooking, preheat the grill to high and toast the bread on both sides. Put the spinach in a saucepan with 1 tablespoon of water and cook over a low heat for about 1 minute until just wilted. Drain the spinach well in a sieve or colander, then press down on the spinach with the back of a wooden spoon to remove as much water as possible.

4   Divide the spinach between the slices of toast and top each one with a poached egg, then spoon the hollandaise sauce over the top. Season to taste with black pepper and serve immediately.

NUTRITION NOTES
PER SERVING

• Calories: 380kcals
• Fat: 19g
• Carbohydrates: 37g

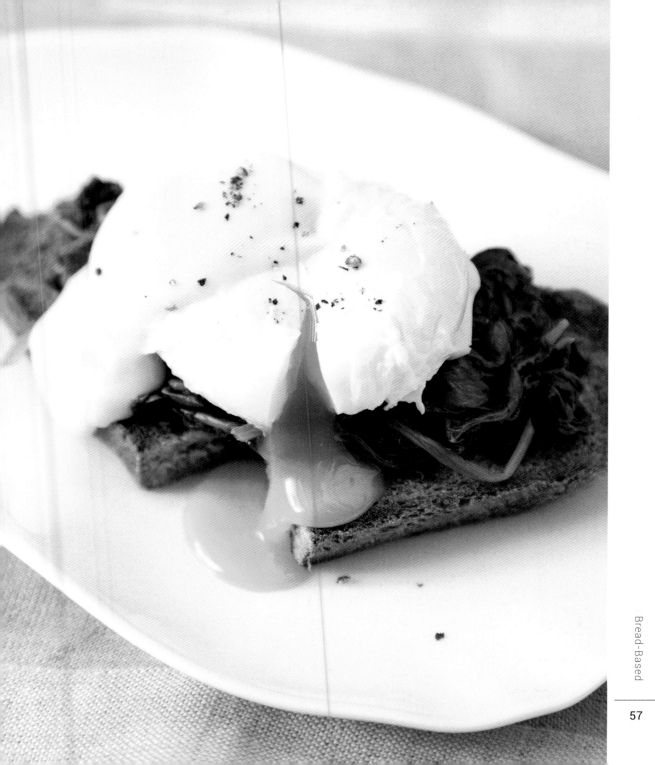

low-calorie cooking oil spray

½ red pepper, deseeded and chopped

¼ red onion, finely chopped

1 garlic clove, crushed

4 mushrooms, thinly sliced

1 tsp dried mixed herbs

2 eggs

2 egg whites

60g/2¼oz mozzarella cheese, diced

4 large tomatoes, halved

2 slices of Almond Rye Bread (see page 48)

a few basil leaves, finely chopped

freshly ground black pepper

Mozzarella & Red Pepper Omelette on Almond Rye with Tomatoes

Serves: 2

Preparation time:
10 minutes, plus
making the bread

Cooking time:
25 minutes

This breakfast is both filling and totally indulgent, with the melted stringy mozzarella cheese giving a chewy texture to every bite.

1 Spray a flameproof non-stick frying pan with a little low-calorie oil spray, add the red pepper, onion and garlic, cover with a lid and cook over a low heat for about 5 minutes, stirring occasionally. Add the mushrooms and cook for a further 3 minutes until softened. Spoon into a bowl and leave to cool for a few minutes. Stir in the mixed herbs, eggs, egg whites, mozzarella and a twist of pepper and mix together well.

2 Return the frying pan to a low heat and coat the pan with a little more of the low-calorie oil spray. Add the egg mixture to the pan, cover and leave to cook for 10–15 minutes, shaking the pan occasionally, until the underside is golden brown and the top is almost set.

3 When it is almost cooked, preheat the grill to high. Put the tomato halves, cut-side up, on the rack and grill for about 4 minutes until browned. Toast the bread on both sides. When the base of the omelette is set, put the omelette in the pan under the grill for about 3 minutes until the top starts to turn golden brown.

4 Divide the omelette in half, sprinkle with the basil and serve with the toast and the grilled tomatoes.

NUTRITION NOTES
PER SERVING
• • • • • • • • • • • • • • • • •
• Calories: 401kcals
• Fat: 14g
• Carbohydrates: 42g

FOR THE WALNUT BREAD

low-calorie cooking oil spray

500g/1lb 2oz/3⅓ cups strong
   wholemeal flour, plus extra
   for dusting

1 tsp fast-action dried yeast

1 tsp ground cinnamon

1 tsp freshly grated nutmeg

2 tbsp chopped walnuts

1 tbsp olive oil

1 tbsp agave nectar

FOR THE CHOCO-NUT SPREAD

2 tbsp peanut butter (no added
   sugar)

1 tbsp chocolate whey protein
   isolate powder

1 tsp agave nectar

Walnut Bread & Choco-Nut Spread

Serves: 2

FOR THE BREAD:
Preparation time:
30 minutes, plus
1½ hours rising

Cooking time:
25 minutes

FOR THE SPREAD:
Preparation time:
5 minutes

Cooking time:
5 minutes

This is a healthy version of that childhood favourite chocolate and nut spread on toast, which may sound naughty but will provide you with good slow-release energy through the morning. To make the loaf in a breadmaker, increase the water to 350ml/12fl oz/1½ cups. Put the liquid ingredients, then the dry ingredients, then the yeast in the breadmaker pan, then simply switch on. Use one slice per serving for this recipe, then enjoy the rest with other breakfasts.

1   To make the bread, lightly grease a large bowl with low-calorie oil spray and line a baking sheet with baking paper.

2   Put the flour, yeast, cinnamon, nutmeg and walnuts in a mixing bowl and stir until combined. Measure 325ml/11fl oz/scant 1⅓ cups of water into a jug, add the oil and agave nectar and mix together. Pour into the flour mixture and combine all the ingredients to form a dough. Turn the dough out on to a lightly floured work surface and knead for about 10 minutes, or until the dough is smooth and elastic. Transfer the kneaded dough to the prepared bowl, cover with cling film and a kitchen towel and leave to rise in a warm place for 1 hour until doubled in size.

3   Knock the air out of the dough, then knead it on a lightly floured work surface for a few minutes. Shape it into a ball and put it on the prepared baking sheet. Cover with a kitchen towel and leave to rise in a warm place for a further 30 minutes.

4   Preheat the oven to 220°C/425°F/gas 7. Remove the kitchen towel and bake the loaf for 25 minutes until golden brown. Transfer to a wire rack and leave to cool.

5   For the chocolate nut spread, put the peanut butter, protein powder and agave nectar in a bowl and blend together well. Preheat the grill to high and toast 2 slices of the bread on both sides. Spread evenly with the chocolate nut spread to serve.

NUTRITION NOTES
PER SERVING
· · · · · · · · · · · · · · · · · · · ·

• Calories: 320kcals
• Fat: 11g
• Carbohydrates: 38g

PER BREAD SLICE
· · · · · · · · · · · · · · · · · · · ·

• Calories: 208kcals
• Fat: 5g
• Carbohydrates: 32g

CHAPTER 3
LUNCH RECIPES

Whether you are at home or at work, and whether you have a relaxed hour or just a rushed 10 minutes for lunch, the recipes in this section offer you a good choice of both quick and simple or more adventurous possibilities. For added convenience, many of them can be prepared the night before to take out with you for your lunch the next day, or you could make enough to reheat portions the following day.

All the lunch recipes are low carbohydrate but have been carefully balanced with good levels of protein, fat and fibre – like this Duck Niçoise Salad (see page 76). As with all of the recipes, as long as you stick to the quantities of each ingredient that are listed, you can then have as much from the free foods list (see page 36) as you like in order to bulk it out into a more substantial meal. And, of course, this is always a good idea as it will make sure you stay full and satisfied for longer.

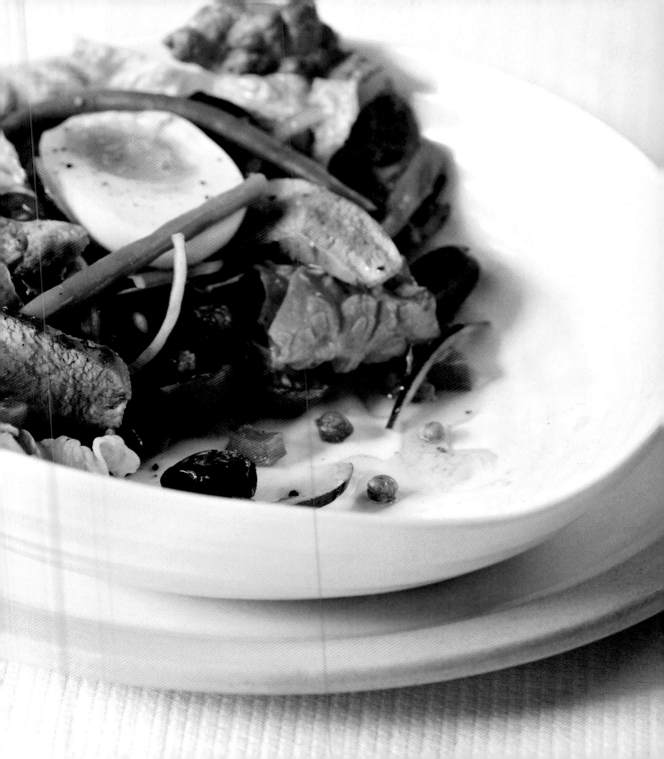

½ onion, finely chopped

2 garlic cloves, crushed

1 leek, trimmed and sliced

2 handfuls of spinach leaves, stems removed

4 slices of bacon, rinded and finely chopped

300ml/10½fl oz/scant 1¼ cups chicken or vegetable stock

2 tbsp double cream

2 egg yolks

freshly ground black pepper

Thick & Creamy Leek & Bacon Soup

Serves: 2

Preparation time: 15 minutes

Cooking time: 40 minutes

This thick, hearty soup is rich and filling and can be made up in large batches to freeze. If you like creamy dishes, then this one is perfect for you.

1 Put the onion and garlic in a large non-stick saucepan over a low heat and add a splash of water to stop the ingredients sticking to the pan. Cook for 5 minutes, stirring occasionally, until softened. Add the leek, spinach and bacon and stir well, then add the stock and season to taste with pepper. Increase the heat and bring to the boil, then turn down the heat to low, cover with a lid and leave to simmer for about 30 minutes, stirring occasionally, until all the ingredients are tender.

2 Remove the soup from the heat and blend to a thick, creamy soup, using a hand-held blender.

3 In a separate bowl, stir together the cream and egg yolks until blended. Stir into the hot soup and serve immediately.

NUTRITION NOTES
PER SERVING
· · · · · · · · · · · · · · · · · ·
• Calories: 391kcals
• Fat: 21g
• Carbohydrates: 14g

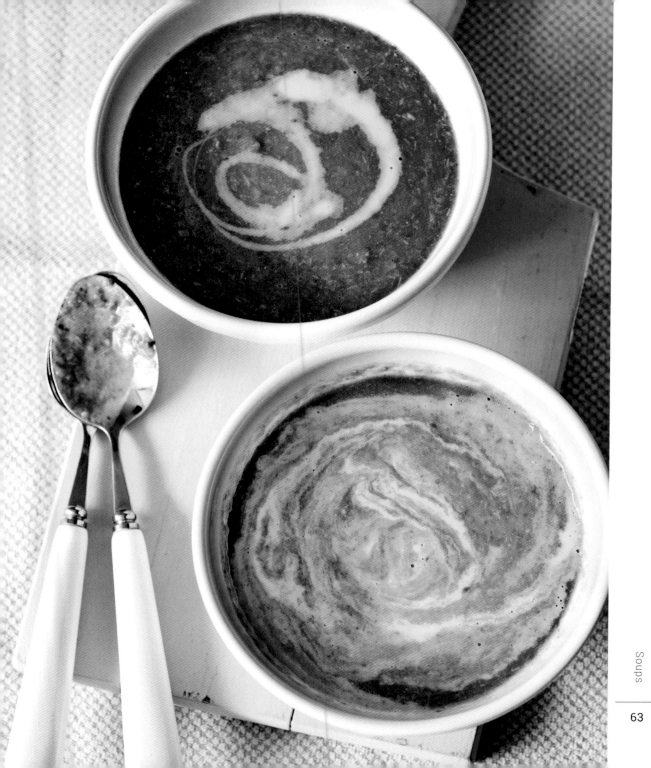

½ onion, finely chopped

4 slices of Parma ham, chopped

200ml/7fl oz/scant 1 cup vegetable
stock

1 large handful of spinach leaves,
stems removed

2 large handfuls of watercress

a pinch of freshly grated nutmeg

2 eggs

1 tbsp crème fraîche

freshly ground black pepper

Watercress Soup with Soft-Boiled Egg & Parma Ham

Serves: 2

Preparation time:
10 minutes

Cooking time:
40 minutes

This is a little lighter and fresher than many soups, making it the perfect post-workout choice, as the antioxidants in watercress aid muscle recovery and counter any cell damage that may be caused by exercise. It is also a great diuretic.

1 Put the onion, Parma ham, stock, spinach, watercress and nutmeg in a large saucepan and season to taste with pepper. Bring to the boil over a medium heat, then turn down the heat to low, cover with a lid and leave to simmer for about 30 minutes until rich and creamy.

2 Meanwhile, put the eggs in a saucepan of cold water. Bring to the boil over a high heat, then turn down the heat to low and leave to simmer for 5 minutes until the eggs are soft-boiled. Remove the eggs from the water using a slotted spoon and leave until cool enough to handle, then peel the eggs and cut into halves.

3 Remove the soup from the heat and stir in the crème fraîche. Float the eggs in the soup and sprinkle with a twist of pepper to serve.

NUTRITION NOTES
PER SERVING
• • • • • • • • • • • • • • • • • •
• Calories: 233kcals
• Fat: 15g
• Carbohydrates: 7g

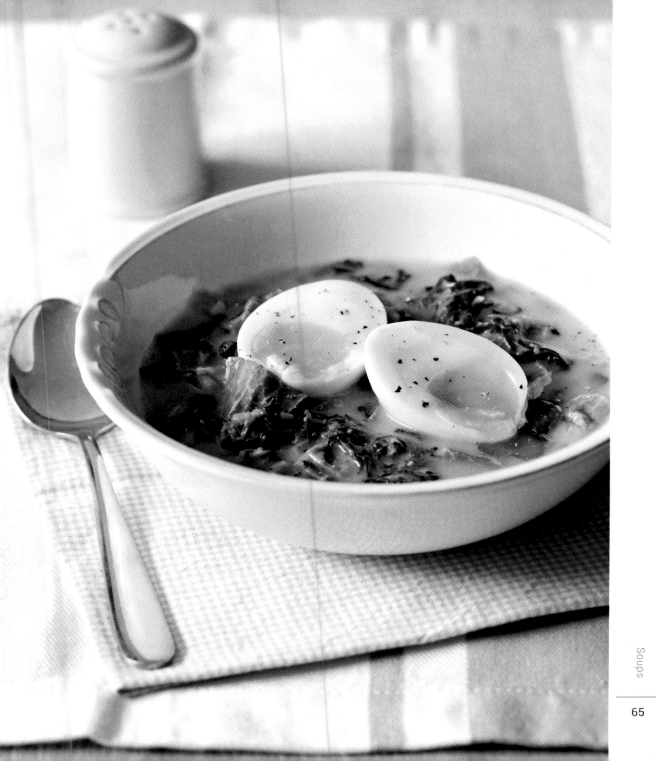

1 large onion, finely chopped

2 garlic cloves, finely chopped

1 celery stick, finely chopped

1 carrot, finely chopped

600ml/21fl oz/scant 2½ cups
   vegetable stock

400g/14oz silken tofu, diced

1 bay leaf

1 small handful of thyme stalks

15 cherry tomatoes

½ tsp stevia powder

½ tsp freshly ground black pepper

200g/7oz passata

1 tbsp balsamic vinegar

2 tbsp double cream

Creamy Tofu Tomato Soup

Serves: 2

Preparation time:
15 minutes

Cooking time:
50 minutes

This may sound strange at first but it is a lovely vegetarian option that actually creates a fantastic, thick, nutritious soup once blended. The inclusion of the protein in the tofu ensures that you feel full all afternoon.

1 Put the onion, garlic, celery and carrot in a large non-stick saucepan over a medium heat. Add a splash of the stock and cook for 5 minutes, stirring continuously, until the vegetables have softened.

2 Add all the remaining ingredients except the cream. Bring to the boil, then turn down the heat to low, cover with a lid and leave to simmer for about 40 minutes until all the vegetables have softened.

3 Remove from the heat and discard the bay leaf and thyme. Stir in the cream, then blend into a smooth soup, using a hand-blender. Serve hot.

NUTRITION NOTES
PER SERVING
• • • • • • • • • • • • • • • • • • •
• Calories: 282kcals
• Fat: 14g
• Carbohydrates: 32g

300g/10½oz chicken livers, trimmed

1 handful of mushrooms, chopped

3 garlic cloves, crushed

¼ onion, finely chopped

1 tsp chopped tarragon leaves

low-calorie cooking oil spray

1 tsp lemon juice

a pinch of stevia powder

2 tbsp cream cheese

2 bay leaves

freshly ground black pepper

FOR THE CRUDITÉS

2 carrots, cut into matchsticks

2 celery sticks, cut into matchsticks

Chicken Liver & Mushroom Pâté with Crudités

Serves: 2

Preparation time:
20 minutes, plus
15 minutes cooling
and 1 hour chilling

Cooking time:
10 minutes

This is a great recipe as it's so versatile. You can serve it as a lunch dish, a starter, or it's perfect if you have a few friends coming over for an afternoon catch-up. Whenever you serve it, you can fill up with plenty of the crudités.

1   Put the chicken livers, mushrooms, garlic, onion and tarragon in a non-stick saucepan over a medium heat and cook for about 10 minutes, stirring occasionally, until the onions are soft and the chicken livers are cooked through. Use a little low-calorie oil spray if the ingredients begin to stick. Remove from the heat and stir through the lemon juice and stevia powder and season to taste with pepper, then leave to cool.

2   Transfer the mixture to a blender or food processor with the cream cheese and blend to a paste. Divide the mixture between two small ramekins, smooth the tops and put a bay leaf in the centre of each one. Cover with cling film and chill in the fridge for at least 1 hour.

3   Serve the pâté with the carrot and celery crudités.

NUTRITION NOTES
PER SERVING
. . . .
• Calories: 188kcals
• Fat: 7g
• Carbohydrates: 3g

360g/12¾oz skinless chicken breast,
    thinly sliced
1 small garlic clove, crushed
¼ red chilli, deseeded and finely
    chopped
juice of ½ lime

1 handful of coriander leaves,
    chopped
1 tbsp soy sauce
½ tsp paprika
1 tsp stevia powder
8 little gem lettuce leaves

FOR THE GUACAMOLE
½ avocado
¼ red onion, finely chopped
1 small garlic clove, crushed
8 cherry tomatoes, finely chopped
1½ tbsp natural yogurt
½ tsp cayenne pepper
freshly ground black pepper

Lime Chicken Strips &
Tomato Guacamole Cups

Serves: 2

Preparation time:
20 minutes, plus
1 hour marinating

Cooking time:
5 minutes

These are a perfect treat on a hot summer's day. Tangy, creamy and crunchy, these delicious morsels will make a refreshing change from your usual bread wrap.

1 Put the chicken in a non-metallic bowl with the garlic, the chilli, lime juice, coriander, soy sauce, paprika and stevia powder. Cover with cling film and leave to marinate in the fridge for at least 1 hour.

2 Transfer the chicken mixture to a non-stick frying pan over a low heat and cook for about 5 minutes, or until the chicken is cooked through, stirring occasionally.

3 Meanwhile, to make the guacamole, peel and pit the avocado, then place the flesh in a bowl and mash with a fork. Mix in the onion, garlic, tomatoes and yogurt, then season to taste with cayenne and black pepper. Mix everything together well.

4 Divide the chicken mixture evenly among the lettuce leaves and top each one with a spoonful of the guacamole to serve.

NUTRITION NOTES
PER SERVING
• • • • • • • • • • • • • • • • •
• Calories: 293kcals
• Fat: 10g
• Carbohydrates: 16g

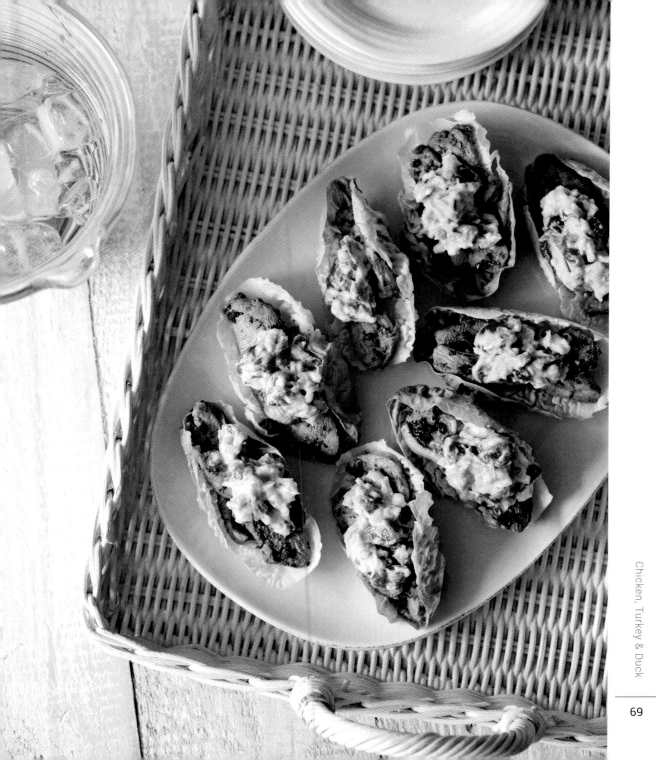

2 skinless chicken breast fillets, each about 180g/6¼oz
2 garlic cloves, crushed
2 tbsp butter

2 tbsp chopped flat-leaf parsley leaves
juice of ½ lemon
freshly ground black pepper

FOR THE GREEN BEAN SALAD
3 spring onions, finely chopped
1 garlic clove, crushed
½ tbsp balsamic vinegar
2 handfuls of green beans
10 cherry tomatoes, halved

Lemon Butter Chicken & Warm Green Bean Salad

Serves: 2

Preparation time:
15 minutes

Cooking time:
20 minutes

This simple but classic Italian-style family dish has a delicious butter sauce that works so perfectly with this elegant green bean salad.

1 Preheat the oven to 180°C/350°F/gas 4. Put two 30cm/12in square pieces of kitchen foil on a baking tray and turn up the edges to make bowl shapes to contain the ingredients. Put a chicken breast in the centre of each piece and top them with the garlic, butter and parsley. Sprinkle over the lemon juice and season with a twist of pepper. Fold the foil loosely over the chicken, then seal the tops to form airtight parcels. Roast for 20 minutes until the chicken is tender and cooked through.

2 Towards the end of the cooking time, put the beans in a steamer, cover with a lid and steam for about 5 minutes until just tender.

3 Meanwhile, to make the salad, put the spring onions, garlic and balsamic vinegar in a non-stick saucepan over a low heat, cover with a lid and cook for about 5 minutes, stirring occasionally, until the onions are softened. Add the green beans and halved tomatoes and cook for a further 2 minutes.

4 Unwrap the chicken and put on top of the salad, then spoon over the cooking juices to serve.

NUTRITION NOTES
PER SERVING
• • • • • • • • • • • • • • • • • •
• Calories: 241kcals
• Fat: 14g
• Carbohydrates: 10g

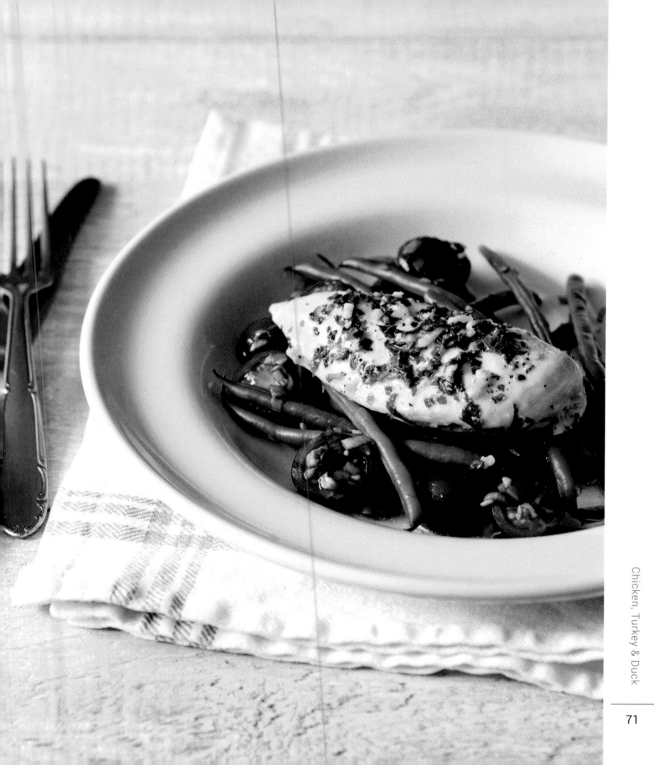

250g/9oz minced turkey

1 egg white

1 tsp chilli powder

1 tsp crushed dried red chilli flakes

1 garlic clove, crushed

2 spring onions, finely chopped

1 tsp dried mixed herbs

½ vegetable stock cube

60g/2¼oz goats' cheese

FOR THE TOMATO AND HERB SALSA

10 cherry tomatoes, finely chopped

1 handful of coriander leaves, finely chopped

½ red onion, finely chopped

¼ red pepper, deseeded and finely chopped

½ tsp stevia powder

juice of ½ lime

freshly ground black pepper

Spicy Turkey Burgers & Goats' Cheese with Tomato & Herb Salsa

Serves: 2

Preparation time: 20 minutes

Cooking time: 15 minutes

If you are craving a classic, unhealthy, greasy burger, just try this recipe and you will be pleasantly surprised by its unique flavours and its healthy, fresh feel. No bun is needed with this delicious lunch.

1 Put the mince, egg white, chilli powder, crushed chilli flakes, garlic, spring onions and mixed herbs in a large bowl and crumble in the stock cube. Using wet hands to stop the mixture sticking to you, mix the ingredients together well, then shape it into 4 equal-sized burgers.

2 Heat a non-stick frying pan over a medium heat, add the burgers and fry for about 5 minutes on each side until slightly browned and cooked through.

3 Meanwhile, mix together all the salsa ingredients. Preheat the grill to high. Once the burgers are cooked, transfer them to the grill, top with the cheese and grill for a few minutes until the cheese has melted.

4 Serve the burgers with the tomato and herb salsa.

NUTRITION NOTES PER SERVING

• Calories: 328kcals

• Fat: 17g

• Carbohydrates: 12g

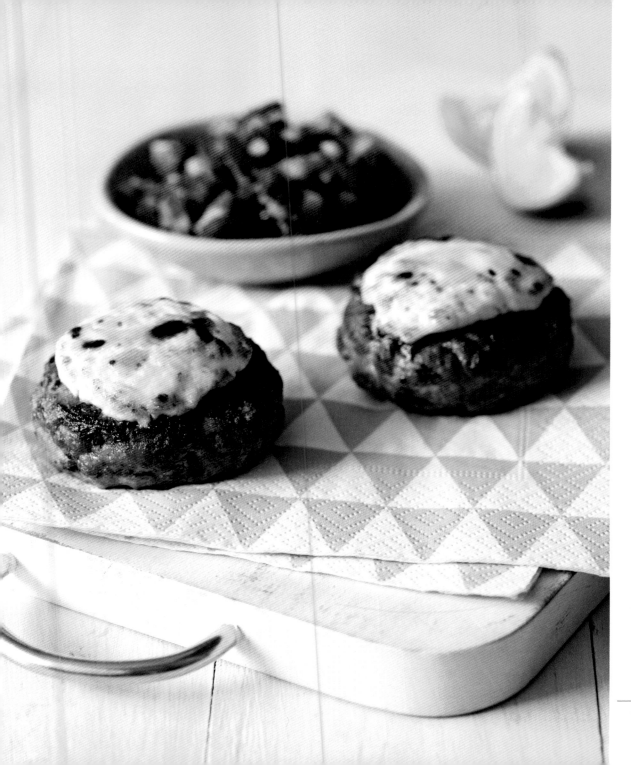

FOR THE CRISPY DUCK

300g/10½oz skinless duck breast, thinly sliced

2 tbsp soy sauce

½ tsp stevia powder

200g/7oz shirataki noodles, drained and rinsed

½ yellow pepper, deseeded and sliced

1 handful of bok choi

¼ small red cabbage, thinly sliced

FOR THE SESAME GINGER DRESSING

2 tbsp sesame oil

1 tbsp white wine vinegar

2 tsp grated root ginger

1 garlic clove, crushed

1 small handful of coriander leaves, finely chopped

1 tsp stevia powder

Duck & Noodle Salad with Sesame Ginger Dressing

Serves: 2

Preparation time: 15 minutes

Cooking time: 10 minutes

I love serving this recipe, especially when I am really hungry. The noodles are made with a special kind of fibre that actually makes you feel fuller for longer, while helping to stabilize blood sugar levels and so prevent those hunger cravings coming back mid-afternoon.

1   Heat a non-stick frying pan over a medium heat and add the duck breast, soy sauce and stevia powder. Cook for 5 minutes, turning regularly, until the duck is cooked through and slightly crisp on the edges. Remove the duck from the pan and leave to one side.

2   Add the shirataki noodles, yellow pepper, bok choi and red cabbage to the pan and cook over a high heat for about 4 minutes, stirring regularly, until heated through and well mixed.

3   To make the dressing, put all the ingredients in a bowl and mix together well.

4   Serve the duck slices on top of the noodle and vegetable mix, drizzled with the sesame ginger dressing.

NUTRITION NOTES
PER SERVING
· · · · · · · · · · · · · · · · · · ·
• Calories: 374kcals
• Fat: 20g
• Carbohydrates: 16g

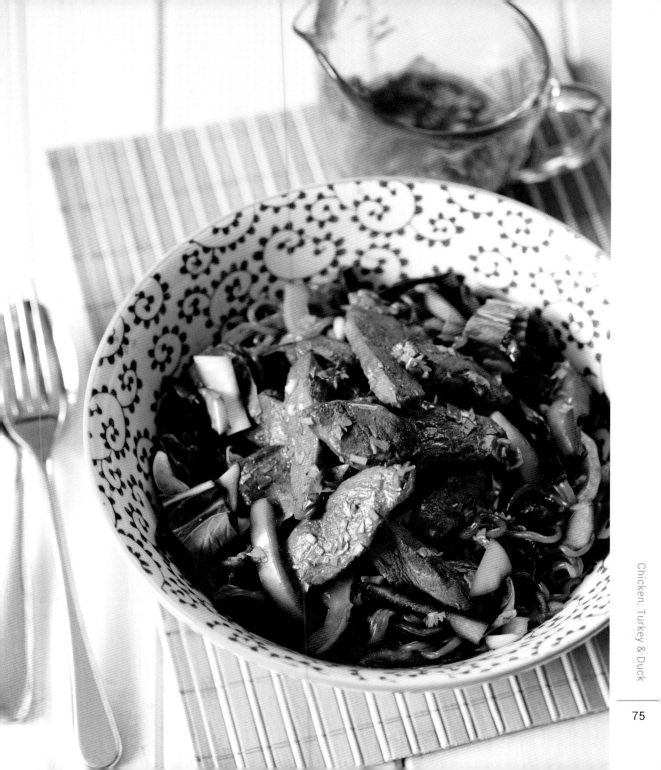

2 tbsp olive oil

1 tsp lemon juice

1 tsp Dijon mustard

200g/7oz skinless duck breast

2 eggs

1 handful of green beans

½ red pepper, deseeded and diced

1 romaine lettuce, torn into pieces

10 cherry tomatoes, halved

½ red onion, thinly sliced

10 black olives, pitted

2 tsp capers

freshly ground black pepper

Duck Niçoise Salad

Serves: 2

Preparation time:
20 minutes, plus
30 minutes marinating

Cooking time:
20 minutes

If you are looking for a change and want to try a slightly more adventurous meal, why not take inspiration from the photograph on page 60 and create my version of the classic Niçoise salad using duck breast.

1   Put the olive oil, lemon juice, mustard and a twist of pepper in a non-metallic bowl and whisk together well. Put the duck in a separate non-metallic bowl and spoon over all but 1 teaspoon of the marinade to coat the duck. Cover with cling film and leave to marinate in the fridge for 30 minutes.

2   Meanwhile, put the eggs in a saucepan of cold water. Bring to the boil over a high heat, then turn down the heat to low and leave to simmer for 5 minutes until the eggs are soft-boiled. Drain and rinse in cold water, then leave to cool completely, peel and cut in half.

3   While the eggs are cooking, put the green beans in a steamer, cover with a lid and steam for about 5 minutes until just tender. Remove from the pan and refresh under cold water.

4   Heat a non-stick frying pan over a medium heat, lift the duck breast out of the marinade, add it to the pan with the red pepper and fry for about 5 minutes on each side, or until cooked through and tender but still slightly pink in the centre.

5   Gently toss together the lettuce, tomatoes, onion, olives and capers. Add the green beans and red pepper and toss again. Slice the duck evenly and add to the salad, top with the eggs, then finish by drizzling the reserved marinade over the salad.

NUTRITION NOTES
PER SERVING
• • • • • • • • • • • • • • • • • •
• Calories: 479kcals
• Fat: 28g
• Carbohydrates: 26g

200g/7oz lean ham, finely chopped

¼ red onion, finely chopped

½ courgette, finely chopped

¼ red pepper, deseeded and finely chopped

1 tsp Dijon mustard

2 eggs, lightly beaten

50g/1¾oz Cheddar cheese, grated

freshly ground black pepper

FOR THE RAINBOW SALAD

2 handfuls of baby spinach leaves

1 cooked beetroot, diced

1 carrot, cut into ribbons using a vegetable peeler

1 tbsp balsamic vinegar

Ham & Courgette Omelette with Rainbow Salad

Serves: 2

Preparation time:
15 minutes, plus
5 minutes cooling

Cooking time:
25 minutes

It makes a good, simple meal choice to whip up a quick omelette to serve with a fresh mixed salad. You can also use any leftover vegetables from the free foods section (see page 36) for this delicious option. Broccoli and over-ripe tomatoes work really well, so they never need to be wasted.

1   Heat a flameproof non-stick frying pan over a low heat, add the ham, onion, courgette and red pepper, cover with a lid and cook for about 5 minutes, stirring occasionally, until the onions are softened. Transfer to a bowl and leave to cool slightly, then add the mustard, eggs and cheese and season to taste with pepper. Mix together well.

2   Reheat the pan over a low heat, then pour the mixture back into the pan, turning the pan so the mixture spreads evenly across the base. Cover with a lid and cook for about 15 minutes, shaking the pan occasionally, until the base is set and the omelette is just cooked through.

3   To make the salad, put the spinach, beetroot and carrot in a bowl, sprinkle over the balsamic vinegar and toss the ingredients together well.

4   Meanwhile, preheat the grill to medium. When the base of the omelette is set, remove the lid and put the omelette in the pan under the grill for about 3 minutes until the top starts to turn golden brown. Cut the omelette in half and serve with the rainbow salad.

NUTRITION NOTES PER SERVING
. . . .
• Calories: 355kcals
• Fat: 17g
• Carbohydrates: 18g

300g/10½oz lamb fillet, cut into
  chunks
2 handfuls of baby spinach leaves
½ red onion, thinly sliced
½ cucumber, chopped

1 tbsp balsamic vinegar
80g/2¾oz feta cheese
2 tbsp pine nuts
freshly ground black pepper

FOR THE CORIANDER YOGURT
  DRESSING
1½ tbsp natural yogurt
1 tbsp finely chopped coriander
  leaves
½ garlic clove, crushed
1 tsp lemon juice

Lamb & Feta Salad with Coriander Yogurt Dressing

Serves: 2

Preparation time:
15 minutes

Cooking time:
5 minutes

This fresh and colourful recipe always reminds me of holidaying in Turkey, but I have added my own special twist to this Middle Eastern dish, using coriander instead of the traditional mint.

1   Heat a non-stick frying pan over a medium heat, add the lamb and cook for about 3 minutes, turning regularly and adding a drop of water, if necessary, to prevent the meat from sticking.

2   Put the spinach, onion, cucumber and balsamic vinegar in a non-metallic bowl. Crumble in the feta and mix well to coat the salad in the vinegar.

3   To make the dressing, put the yogurt in a small, non-metallic bowl and mix in the coriander, garlic and lemon juice.

4   Top the salad with the lamb pieces, sprinkle with the pine nuts and season with pepper, then serve with a dollop of the dressing.

NUTRITION NOTES
PER SERVING
· · · · · · · · · · · · · · · · ·
• Calories: 375kcals
• Fat: 23g
• Carbohydrates: 15g

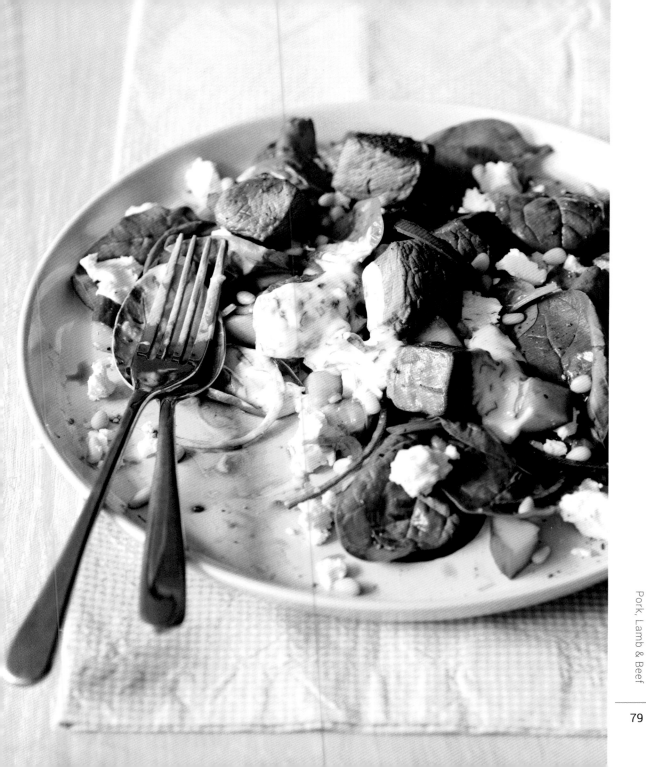

½ onion, finely chopped

1 garlic clove, crushed

1 tsp ground cumin

1 tsp chilli powder

1 tsp ground coriander

½ tsp cayenne pepper

200g/7oz minced lamb

1 egg white

1 yellow pepper, deseeded and cut
into large chunks

1 courgette, cut into chunky slices

low-calorie cooking oil spray

2 handfuls of rocket leaves

freshly ground black pepper

FOR THE MUSTARD DIPPING SAUCE

70ml/2¼fl oz/scant ⅓ cup crème
fraîche

½ tbsp wholegrain mustard

1 tsp agave nectar

1 tsp lemon juice

a pinch of cayenne pepper

Spicy Lamb Skewers with Mustard Dipping Sauce

Serves: 2

Preparation time:
20 minutes, plus
40 minutes cooling
and chilling

Cooking time:
25 minutes

These skewers are great for sharing, and it's fun to let everyone get involved with helping to prepare them, too.

1   Heat a non-stick frying pan over a low heat, add the onion, garlic, cumin, chilli, coriander and cayenne and season to taste with black pepper. Cover with a lid and cook over a low heat for about 5 minutes, stirring occasionally, until the onions have softened. You may want to add a drop of water to prevent the ingredients from sticking. Remove from the heat and leave to cool.

2   Transfer the vegetables to a large bowl and add the lamb mince and egg white. Using wet hands to stop the mixture sticking to you, mix all the ingredients together well, then cover with cling film and chill in the fridge for 30 minutes.

3   Preheat the grill to medium. Divide the lamb mixture, the yellow pepper and courgette into four and grease four metal skewers with low-calorie oil spray. Take a small handful of the lamb mixture and form it into a ball around one end of the first skewer. Thread a piece of yellow pepper, then a piece of courgette on to the skewer, and repeat until you have used a quarter of the ingredients. Repeat with the remaining skewers. Grill the skewers for about 20 minutes, rotating frequently, until cooked through.

4   To make the dipping sauce, mix together all the ingredients with a twist of black pepper until well blended. Serve the skewers on top of the rocket with a spoonful of the dipping sauce.

**NUTRITION NOTES
PER SERVING**

• Calories: 414kcals

• Fat: 29g

• Carbohydrates: 17g

2 tbsp sesame oil

3 spring onions, chopped

½ red pepper, deseeded and sliced

1 carrot, cut into ribbons using a
  vegetable peeler

1 handful of baby broccoli florets

1 handful of bok choi leaves

200g/7oz lean steak, thinly sliced

2 garlic cloves, crushed

1 tsp grated root ginger

5 sweet basil leaves, finely chopped

1 tsp crushed dried red chilli flakes

1 tbsp soy sauce

60ml/2fl oz/¼ cup vegetable stock

1 tsp stevia powder

juice of ½ lime

freshly ground black pepper

1½ tbsp natural yogurt, to serve

Beef Stir-Fry

Serves: 2

Preparation time:
20 minutes

Cooking time:
10 minutes

This dish is really simple to prepare and works with chicken, turkey, tender lamb or pork substituted for the beef, if you prefer. If you want to bulk it out even more, you can also try adding some shirataki noodles.

1 Heat the oil in a non-stick wok or large frying pan over a high heat, add the spring onions, red pepper, carrot, broccoli and bok choi. Stir-fry over a high heat for about 3 minutes until hot and well blended.

2 Add the steak, garlic, ginger, basil, crushed chilli flakes, soy sauce, stock, stevia powder and lime juice. Continue to cook, uncovered, over a high heat for about 5 minutes, stirring and tossing, until the meat and vegetables are cooked through.

3 Season to taste with pepper and serve topped with a spoonful of yogurt.

NUTRITION NOTES
PER SERVING
· · · · · · · · · · · · · · · · ·
• Calories: 399kcals
• Fat: 21g
• Carbohydrates: 22g

Pork, Lamb & Beef

200g/7oz lean steak, thinly sliced

1 tbsp soy sauce

1 tsp grated root ginger

1 garlic clove, crushed

1 tsp crushed dried red chilli flakes

1 tsp chilli powder

1 tsp stevia powder

juice of ½ lime

2 tbsp sesame seeds

1 handful of coriander leaves, chopped

1½ tbsp natural yogurt

FOR THE ASIAN SALAD

1 carrot, finely chopped

3 spring onions, finely chopped

½ cucumber, finely chopped

6 cherry tomatoes, finely chopped

2 handfuls of romaine lettuce leaves, torn into pieces

Sesame Beef with Asian Salad

Serves: 2

Preparation time:
15 minutes, plus
1 hour marinating

Cooking time:
10 minutes

Why not try something different for lunch today? Give a traditional salad a fantastic twist for a change with this Asian-style combination of flavours. It is extremely flavoursome with a nice, spicy kick!

1   Put the steak in a non-metallic bowl and add the soy sauce, ginger, garlic, crushed chilli flakes, chilli powder, stevia powder and lime juice. Mix together well, cover with cling film and leave to marinate in the fridge for 1 hour.

2   Heat a non-stick frying pan over a medium heat, add the steak with its marinade, cover with a lid and cook for about 3–6 minutes, stirring occasionally, until the steak is just browned. Add the sesame seeds and coriander and cook for a further 1 minute, stirring to coat the steak in the juices.

3   In a separate bowl, mix together the carrot, spring onions, cucumber, tomatoes and lettuce. Top the salad with the steak and serve with a dollop of yogurt.

NUTRITION NOTES
PER SERVING
. . . .
• Calories: 352kcals
• Fat: 17g
• Carbohydrates: 19g

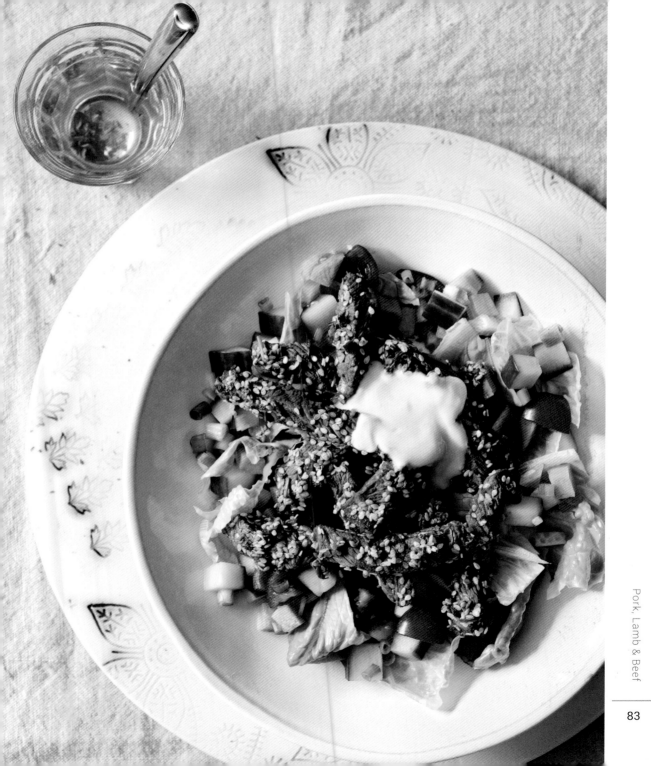

2 mackerel fillets, each about 100g/3½oz

1 large tomato, sliced

½ red pepper, deseeded and chopped

½ red onion, chopped

1 courgette, chopped

1 tbsp lemon juice

1 handful of parsley leaves, chopped

1 bay leaf, torn into quarters

2 handfuls of rocket leaves

freshly ground black pepper

FOR THE GARLIC PESTO

1 handful of basil leaves

1 tbsp lemon juice

2 tbsp olive oil

1 garlic clove, crushed

Baked Mackerel with Vegetables & Garlic Pesto

Serves: 2

Preparation time: 20 minutes

Cooking time: 25 minutes

This is a really fresh, healthy dish but probably not recommended for a first date! The strong garlic pesto perfectly complements the flavour of the mackerel.

1 Preheat the oven to 180°C/350°F/gas 4. Put the mackerel in a baking tin and put a line of tomato slices on top to cover the fish. Sprinkle with the red pepper, onion and courgette, then drizzle over the lemon juice. Sprinkle with the parsley and season to taste with pepper, then add the pieces of bay leaf. Bake for 25 minutes.

2 Meanwhile, to make the garlic pesto, put the basil leaves, lemon juice, olive oil, garlic and 1 tablespoon of water in a small blender or food processor and blend to a smooth paste.

3 Top the rocket leaves with the mackerel and vegetables, then drizzle over the garlic pesto to serve.

NUTRITION NOTES
PER SERVING
• • • • • • • • • • • • • • • • • • •
• Calories: 369kcals
• Fat: 22g
• Carbohydrates: 17g

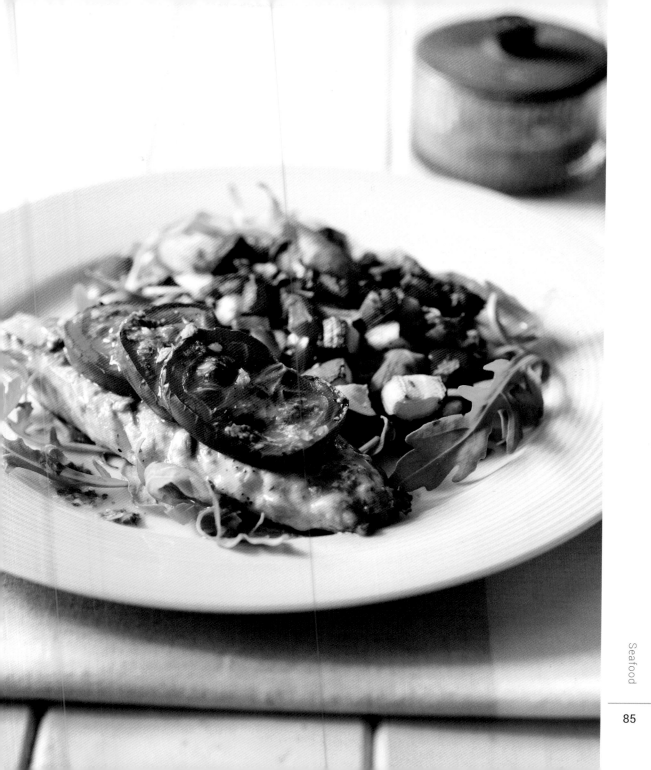

200g/7oz smoked salmon

2 heaped tbsp cream cheese

1 handful of chive stalks, finely
 chopped

1 garlic clove, crushed

juice of ½ lemon

2 handfuls of watercress

freshly ground black pepper

FOR THE CUCUMBER DILL SALAD

½ cucumber, thinly sliced

¼ red onion, thinly sliced

1 handful of dill leaves, finely
 chopped

1 tbsp capers

Smoked Salmon Parcels with Cucumber Dill Salad

Serves: 2

Preparation time:
20 minutes, plus
1 hour chilling

Another stylish summer recipe, this is ideal for a light lunch. Try making this if you have invited friends over – this lovely dish will surely impress them.

1   Line two ramekin dishes with the salmon so that it covers the base and sides and hangs over the edges. Chop any remaining salmon finely. Put the cream cheese, chives, garlic and lemon juice in a non-metallic bowl and season with pepper. Add any chopped salmon and mix together well.

2   Spoon the mixture evenly into the centre of the ramekins and smooth it down, then wrap the loose edges of the salmon over the top to contain the filling into a parcel. Cover with cling film and chill in the fridge for 1 hour.

3   To make the salad, mix together the cucumber and onion, then sprinkle with the dill and capers. Remove the salmon parcels from the ramekins, put on top of the cucumber salad and finish with a handful of watercress.

NUTRITION NOTES
PER SERVING
• • • • • • • • • • • • • • • • • •

• Calories: 269kcals

• Fat: 16g

• Carbohydrates: 12g

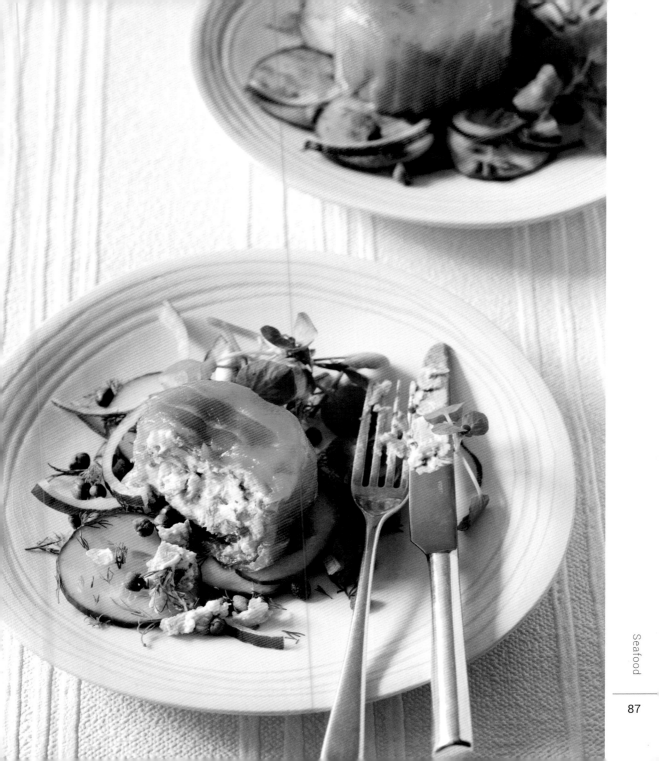

FOR THE BEETROOT AND AVOCADO SALAD

1 raw beetroot

½ avocado

2 handfuls of rocket leaves

FOR THE LEMON AND CHILLI SARDINES

1 tbsp lemon juice

1 garlic clove, crushed

1 tsp crushed dried red chilli flakes

1 small handful of coriander leaves, finely chopped

320g/11¼oz fresh sardine fillets

8 cherry tomatoes, halved

1 tbsp balsamic vinegar

freshly ground black pepper

Lemon & Chilli Sardines with Beetroot & Avocado Salad

Serves: 2

Preparation time: 15 minutes, plus 1 hour chilling

Cooking time: 1¼ hours

Sardines just aren't eaten often enough as far as I'm concerned. They are one of the most concentrated sources of beneficial omega-3 and so are incredibly good for lowering your cholesterol levels. For speed, you can use a cooked beetroot, in which case, simply trim and dice at step 1.

1 To cook the beetroot, wash and trim the stalk slightly. Submerge in a saucepan of boiling water, then turn down the heat, cover with a lid and leave to simmer for about 1 hour until tender. Drain and leave to cool, then peel and dice.

2 Meanwhile, to make the marinade, mix together the lemon juice, garlic, crushed chilli flakes and coriander in a non-metallic bowl. Add the sardines, cover with cling film and chill in the fridge for 1 hour.

3 Preheat the grill to low. Put the tomatoes in a small roasting tin and sprinkle lightly with the balsamic vinegar. Grill for about 5 minutes. Turn the grill to high, then grill the sardines for a few minutes on each side until cooked through, turning carefully.

4 Peel, pit and dice the avocado, then immediately toss together with the beetroot and season with a twist of pepper. Sprinkle over a bed of rocket, top with the sardines and tomatoes, then finish with another twist of pepper to taste.

NUTRITION NOTES PER SERVING

• Calories: 292kcals

• Fat: 8g

• Carbohydrates: 14g

400g/14oz firm tofu, diced

2 egg whites

1 garlic clove, crushed

3 spring onions, chopped

1 carrot, cut into ribbons using a
vegetable peeler

1 handful of bean sprouts

1 courgette, cut into ribbons using a
vegetable peeler

1 tbsp vegetarian not-fish sauce or
Thai fish sauce

1 tbsp soy sauce

1 tsp stevia powder

1 tsp crushed dried red chilli flakes

200g/7oz shirataki noodles, drained
and rinsed

1 lime

1 handful of coriander leaves,
finely chopped

40g/1½oz/¼ cup raw unsalted
peanuts, chopped

Peanut & Tofu Pad Thai

Serves: 2

Preparation time:
20 minutes

Cooking time:
10 minutes

Full of protein, this popular Thai classic has the added benefit of being super healthy. Obviously, vegetarians would not use traditional Thai fish sauce but there are vegetarian versions made with wakame seaweed, often called not-fish sauce. To make the recipe gluten free, substitute a gluten-free soy sauce for the traditional soy sauce.

1 Put the tofu in a non-stick wok or large saucepan over a medium heat and cook for a few minutes until golden, tossing gently, then remove from the pan.

2 Add the egg whites to the pan and cook for 1 minute, stirring continuously. Add the garlic, spring onions, carrot, bean sprouts and courgette and cook for a further 1 minute. Return the tofu to the pan and add the not-fish sauce, soy sauce, stevia powder, crushed chilli flakes and shirataki noodles. Cook over a medium heat for about 5 minutes, stirring occasionally, until cooked through.

3 Cut the lime in half and cut one half into wedges. Remove the pan from the heat and stir in the coriander and the juice of the half lime. Sprinkle with the peanuts and serve with the remaining lime wedges.

NUTRITION NOTES
PER SERVING
· · · · · · · · · · · · · · · · ·

• Calories: 334kcals
• Fat: 14g
• Carbohydrates: 24g

Seafood / Vegetarian

4 red peppers, deseeded and halved
   vertically
400g/14oz firm tofu, finely chopped
1 garlic clove, finely chopped
¼ red onion, chopped

4 mushrooms, chopped
1 tsp chopped oregano leaves
1 tbsp passata
1 tsp stevia powder
½ tsp smoked paprika

80g/2¾oz mozzarella cheese, grated
freshly ground black pepper
2 large handfuls of mixed salad
   leaves, to serve

Tofu-Stuffed Red Peppers

Serves: 2

Preparation time:
15 minutes, plus
4 minutes soaking

Cooking time:
35 minutes

Another great vegetarian choice for a filling lunch, the sweetness of the peppers works wonderfully with the creamy melted cheese.

1   Preheat the oven to 180°C/350°F/gas 4. Put the red peppers in a bowl, cover with boiling water and leave to stand for about 4 minutes until softened slightly. Drain and pat dry on kitchen paper.

2   Heat a non-stick frying pan over a low heat and add the tofu, garlic, onion, mushrooms, oregano, passata, stevia powder and paprika, then season to taste with pepper. Stir until heated through, then leave to simmer over a low heat for about 10 minutes until the onions and garlic have softened, adding a splash of water, if necessary, if the ingredients begin to stick. Remove from the heat and leave to cool for a few minutes, then stir in the mozzarella and mix together well.

3   Put the red peppers, skin-side down, in a baking tray and spoon the mixture evenly into the peppers, packing it into the centre of each one. Bake for about 20 minutes until the red peppers are tender and the topping is bound by the melted mozzarella. Serve hot with the mixed salad leaves.

NUTRITION NOTES
PER SERVING
• • • • • • • • • • • • • • • • • •

• Calories: 378kcals
• Fat: 17g
• Carbohydrates: 24g

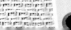

60g/2¼oz halloumi cheese, patted dry and cut into 6 pieces

1 small garlic clove, crushed

2 large pinches of dried oregano

1 tbsp finely grated lemon zest

½ tsp crushed dried red chilli flakes

low-calorie cooking oil spray

1 red pepper, deseeded and sliced

2 tbsp balsamic vinegar

2 tsp agave nectar

6 iceberg lettuce leaves

2 tbsp tahini

4 tbsp lemon juice

Marinated Halloumi & Caramelized Red Pepper Wraps

Serves: 2

Preparation time:
10 minutes, plus
at least 2 hours
marinating

Cooking time:
5 minutes

These crunchy wraps have a fresh, sweet and salty taste and are perfect to take to work for your lunch break. You may want to keep the lettuce separate and assemble when you are ready to eat them.

1   Put the halloumi, garlic, oregano, lemon zest and crushed chilli flakes in a non-metallic bowl. Lightly mist with low-calorie oil spray and stir well, making sure the halloumi is well coated. Cover with cling film and leave to marinate in the fridge for 2–3 hours or you can leave it overnight.

2   Heat a non-stick frying pan over a medium-high heat. Add the halloumi and cook for about 5 minutes until golden, turning regularly.

3   Meanwhile, heat another non-stick frying pan over a medium-high heat. Add the red pepper, balsamic vinegar and agave nectar and cook for 4–5 minutes, stirring occasionally, until the red pepper has softened.

4   Put the lettuce leaves on a chopping board and evenly spoon the halloumi and red pepper into the centre of each leaf. Whisk the tahini and lemon juice together with 2 tablespoons of boiling water in a small bowl. Evenly drizzle the dressing over the top of the fillings, then roll up the lettuce leaves and serve immediately.

NUTRITION NOTES
PER SERVING
· · · · · · · · · · · · · · · · · ·
• Calories: 205kcals
• Fat: 8g
• Carbohydrates: 24g

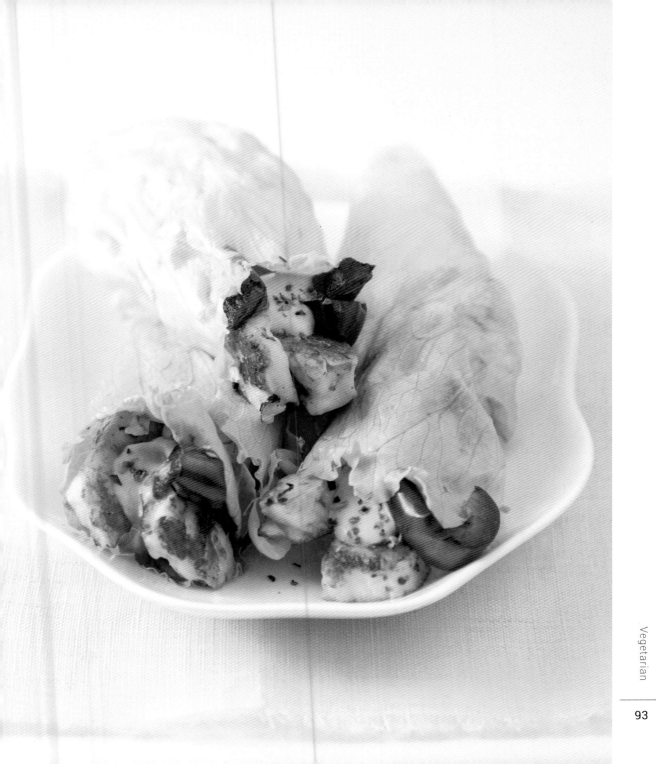

1½ tbsp butter

65g/2¼oz/⅔ cup ground almonds

½ red onion, thinly sliced

1 garlic clove, crushed

1 tbsp balsamic vinegar

1 tsp agave nectar

6 asparagus tips, trimmed

1 egg

1½ tbsp natural yogurt

2 tsp Dijon mustard

freshly ground black pepper

2 handfuls of mixed salad leaves
    and 6 cherry tomatoes, cut into
    wedges, to serve

Red Onion Tartlets with Baked Asparagus

Serves: 2

Preparation time:
**10 minutes, plus
15 minutes cooling**

Cooking time:
25 minutes

My mum loves this dish so I always make sure to cook her a supply for the freezer when I visit. Sweet, buttery and totally gluten-free, it is so delicious.

1   Preheat the oven to 180°C/350°F/gas 4. Heat the butter in a small non-stick saucepan over a low heat until melted, then stir in the ground almonds and mix together well. Press the mixture into two sections of a muffin tin and pat down with your fingers into the bottom and a little way up the sides to create a base for the tartlets. Bake for 5 minutes, then remove from the oven.

2   Put the onion, garlic, balsamic vinegar and agave nectar in a non-stick saucepan over a low heat and cook for a few minutes until softened. Spoon the mixture into a bowl and leave to cool.

3   While it is cooling, cut a 40cm/16in square of kitchen foil and put the asparagus tips on top. Bring the edges up over the asparagus to make a loose pouch and seal the edges tightly. Put on the muffin tin next to the tarts.

4   Stir the egg, yogurt and mustard into the onion mixture and season to taste with pepper. Spoon into the baked tartlet bases and return them to the oven, with the asparagus, for 20 minutes until the centres of the tarts are just firm and the tops are very lightly golden. Leave to cool a little in the tin.

5   Top the tartlets with the asparagus and serve with the salad leaves scattered with tomato wedges and seasoned with a little more black pepper.

NUTRITION NOTES
PER SERVING
....

• Calories: 372kcals
• Fat: 29g
• Carbohydrates: 20g

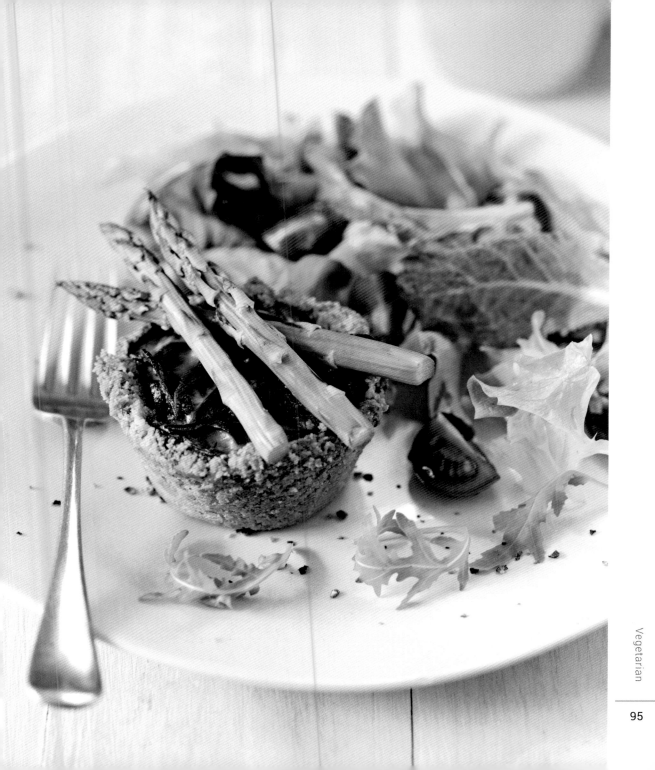

CHAPTER 4
DINNER RECIPES

Luckily, some of us have a little more time in the evenings to prepare a good home-cooked meal, although I appreciate that a lot of people – including most working mothers – may have less time to work with. The following recipes include a mix of quick and simple dishes and some that are more adventurous – like this Haddock with Spiced Cayenne Peanuts (see page 136). They can all be shared by the whole family just by adding some carbohydrate for children and non-dieters – all the recipes work well with rice, pasta or potatoes, although, of course, these accompaniments are not for you. But you do have the choice to add as much from the free foods section (see page 36) as you like in order to bulk out the meal and make sure you are not hungry in the evening.

There is a good selection of meat, fish and vegetarian recipes so make sure you mix it up and try not to have more than one of the red meat dishes per week. The best options for optimal health and weight loss will always be the fish dishes, so try to serve fish dishes regularly.

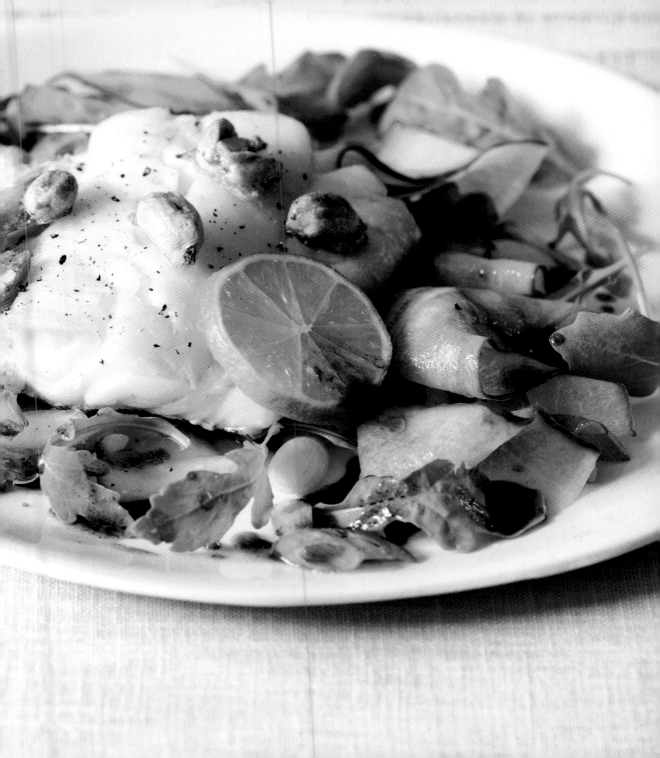

300ml/10½fl oz/scant 1¼ cups hot
   chicken stock
¼ tsp saffron threads, crushed
½ onion, finely chopped
2 garlic cloves, crushed
1 tsp ground ginger
1 tsp ground cumin

1 tsp ground cinnamon
1 tbsp tomato purée
2 skinless chicken breasts, each
   about 180g/6¼oz
30g/1oz/scant ¼ cup almonds,
   roughly chopped
15 olives, pitted and chopped

½ tbsp lemon juice
1 large handful of coriander leaves,
   chopped
freshly ground black pepper
mixed salad leaves, to serve

Rich Almond Chicken Tagine

Serves: 2

Preparation time:
20 minutes

Cooking time:
30 minutes

With its circulation-boosting blend of warming spices, this rich and flavoursome dish makes a great winter meal. It also works well with beef or white fish instead of the chicken if you want a change. I generally use green olives.

1   Put the hot stock in a bowl, add the saffron and leave to infuse.

2   Meanwhile, put the onion and 1 tablespoon of water in a large heavy-based saucepan over a medium heat and cook for a few minutes until softened. Add the garlic, ginger, cumin and cinnamon, season to taste with pepper and cook for a further 2 minutes. Add the stock, tomato purée, chicken, almonds, olives and lemon juice and bring to the boil. Turn down the heat to low, cover with a lid and leave to simmer for about 20 minutes, stirring occasionally, until the chicken is cooked through and tender.

3   Remove from the heat and stir well. Sprinkle with the chopped coriander and serve with a mixed green salad.

NUTRITION NOTES
PER SERVING
● ● ● ● ● ● ● ● ● ● ● ● ● ● ●
• Calories: 361kcals
• Fat: 14g
• Carbohydrates: 12g

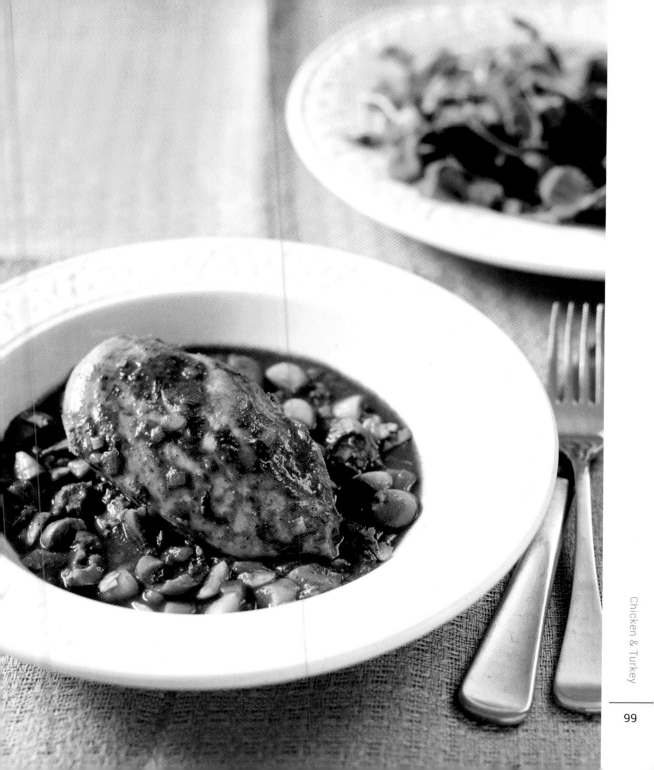

2 handfuls of baby spinach leaves

2 skinless chicken breast fillets,
    each about 180g/6¼oz

60g/2¼oz soft goats' cheese

1 tsp finely chopped tarragon leaves

4 slices of Parma ham

6–8 large cauliflower florets

200g/7oz asparagus tips, trimmed,
    or other vegetables

freshly ground black pepper

Parma Ham-Wrapped Chicken with Cauliflower Purée

Serves: 2

Preparation time:
15 minutes

Cooking time:
20 minutes

This beautifully presented dish looks almost too good to eat! The cauliflower purée offers a great substitute for a high-carbohydrate mashed potato plus it's loaded with B vitamins to help energy release.

1   Preheat the oven to 200°C/400°F/gas 6. Put the spinach in a saucepan with 1 tablespoon of water and cook over a low heat for about 1 minute until just wilted. Drain the spinach well in a sieve or colander, then press down on the spinach with the back of a wooden spoon to remove as much water as possible.

2   Put the chicken breasts on a chopping board and cut each one open horizontally along the middle, keeping them 'hinged' along one edge. To make the stuffing, mix together the goats' cheese, tarragon and wilted spinach in a bowl. Divide the stuffing mixture between the chicken breasts, spreading it across the cut sides of each one. Season to taste with pepper and enclose the stuffing. Tightly wrap 2 slices of Parma ham around each chicken breast to hold the stuffing in place. Transfer the wrapped chicken to a non-stick baking sheet and bake for 15–20 minutes until the juices run clear when the meat is pierced with the tip of a sharp knife or skewer.

3   Meanwhile, put the cauliflower florets in a steamer, cover with a lid and steam for about 20 minutes until very soft. Add the asparagus after 10 minutes so that they finish cooking at the same time.

4   Transfer the steamed cauliflower to a food processor, season with pepper and process to a smooth purée. Divide the cauliflower purée, chicken and steamed asparagus into two equal portions and serve hot.

NUTRITION NOTES
PER SERVING
••••••••••••••••

• Calories: 397kcals
• Fat: 14g
• Carbohydrates: 8g

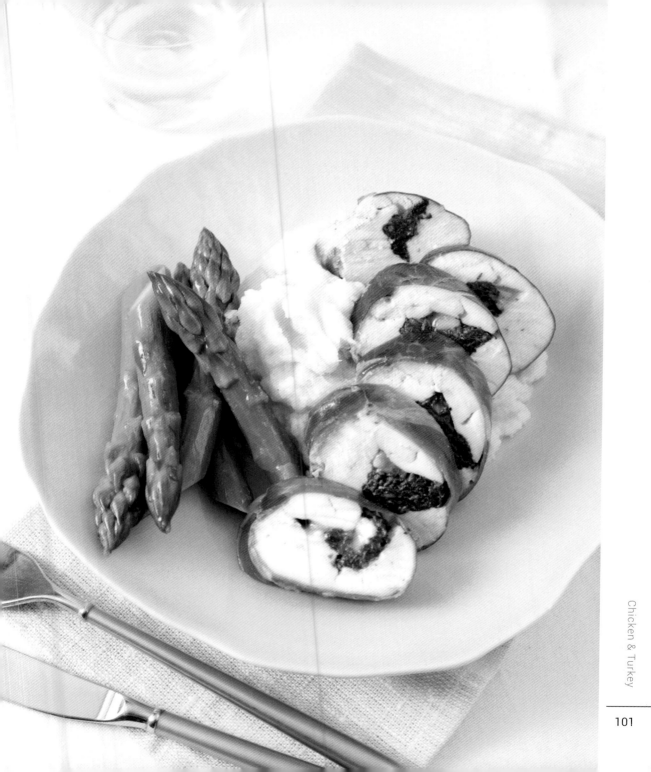

½ onion, finely chopped

150ml/5fl oz/scant ⅔ cup chicken stock

1 garlic clove, crushed

1 tsp grated root ginger

1 tsp ground cumin

1 tsp ground coriander

½ tsp ground cinnamon

1 tsp chilli powder

1 tsp crushed dried red chilli flakes

360g/12¾oz skinless chicken breast, diced

15 cashew nuts, chopped

1 bay leaf

8 cherry tomatoes

2 tbsp double cream

1 tsp stevia powder

200g/7oz green beans and broccoli

1 handful of coriander leaves, chopped

freshly ground black pepper

FOR THE CAULIFLOWER RICE

200g/7oz cauliflower florets

low-calorie cooking oil spray

Chicken & Cashew Nut Korma

Serves: 2

Preparation time: 15 minutes

Cooking time: 30 minutes

Forget your Friday night Indian take-away and give this healthy version a try instead. Although it is not served with the customary rice, it is still thick, creamy and authentically delicious.

1 Put the onion and 1 tablespoon of the stock in a heavy-based, non-stick saucepan over a medium heat and cook for 2 minutes. Add the garlic, ginger and spices, season to taste with pepper and cook for 1–2 minutes. Add the chicken, cashews and bay leaf and cook for a few minutes until the chicken starts to brown slightly. Add the remaining stock and bring to the boil. Turn down the heat to low and leave to simmer gently for about 15 minutes.

2 Add the tomatoes, cream and stevia powder, return to the boil, cover with a lid and leave to simmer for a further 5–10 minutes until the chicken is cooked through, stirring occasionally.

3 Meanwhile, put the beans and broccoli in a steamer, cover with a lid and steam for about 6 minutes until just tender.

4 Put the cauliflower florets in a blender or food processor and blend until finely chopped. Heat a dry, non-stick frying pan over a low heat, spray lightly with low-calorie oil spray, then add the cauliflower and shake over a low heat for a few minutes until just tender.

5 Remove the curry from the heat, add the chopped coriander and stir together. Serve with the steamed green beans, broccoli and cauliflower rice.

NUTRITION NOTES
PER SERVING
• • • • • • • • • • • • • • • •
• Calories: 404kcals
• Fat: 17g
• Carbohydrates: 18g

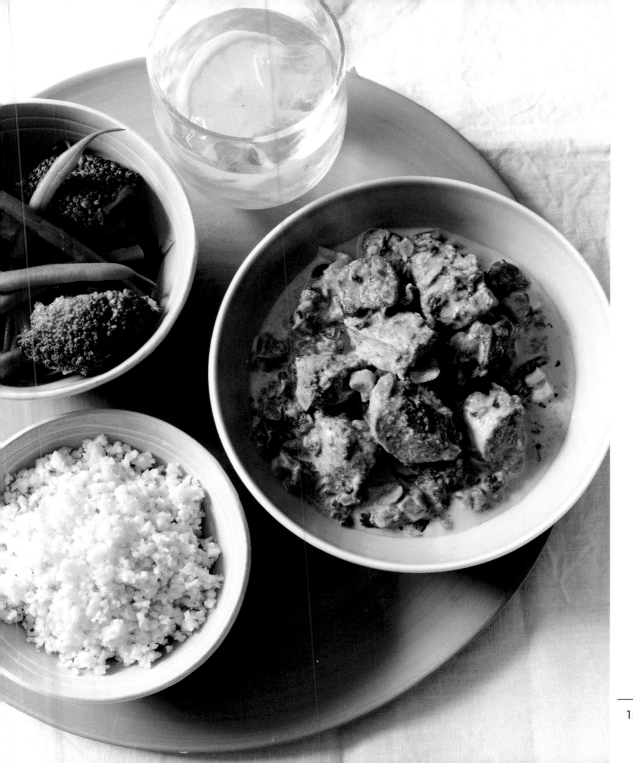

360g/12¾oz skinless chicken breast, thinly sliced

½ onion, finely chopped

35g/1¼oz/scant ¼ cup almonds, roughly chopped

175g/6oz button mushrooms, sliced

1 tsp chopped dill leaves

1 large handful of spinach leaves, stems removed

3 tbsp double cream

1 tbsp wholegrain mustard

1 tsp white wine vinegar

½ tsp white pepper

200g/7oz green beans

Chicken & Mushrooms in an Almond & Mustard Sauce

Serves: 2

Preparation time: 15 minutes

Cooking time: 10 minutes

Beautifully creamy and tangy, this sauce really livens up the chicken and makes for an all-round nutritious and delicious meal.

1 Put the chicken and onion in a non-stick saucepan over a low heat, cover with a lid and cook for about 3 minutes, shaking the pan occasionally, until the chicken is just beginning to brown.

2 Add the almonds, mushrooms and dill to the chicken and cook for a further 2 minutes. Add the spinach, cream, mustard, wine vinegar and white pepper, stir well, then cover and cook over a low heat for a further 5 minutes until the chicken is tender and cooked through.

3 Meanwhile, put the beans in a steamer, cover with a lid and steam for 5 minutes until just tender. Serve with the chicken.

NUTRITION NOTES PER SERVING
••••••••••••••••
• Calories: 450kcals
• Fat: 24g
• Carbohydrates: 16g

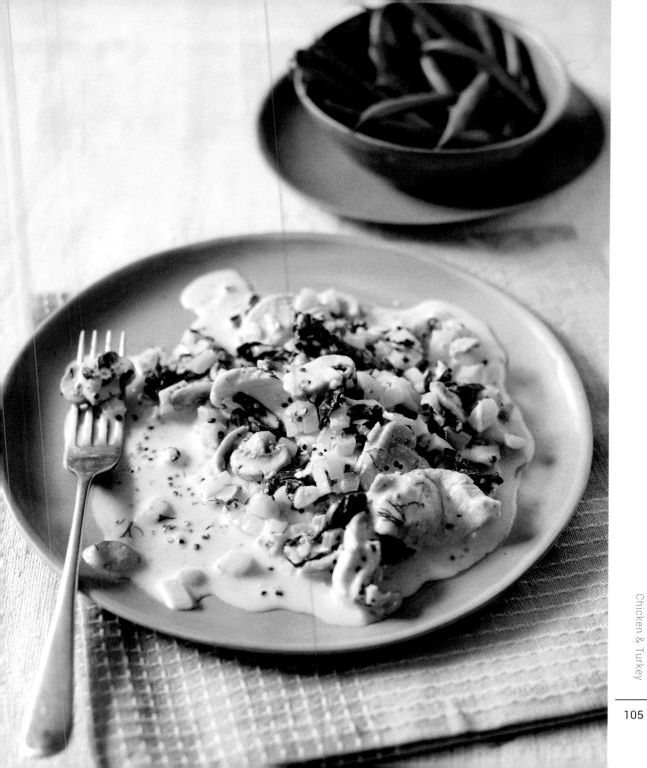

½ red pepper, deseeded and
   thinly sliced

8 cherry tomatoes, halved

1 tbsp balsamic vinegar

60ml/2fl oz/¼ cup chicken stock

1 tsp chilli powder

1 tsp crushed dried red chilli flakes

1 small handful of coriander leaves,
   finely chopped

360g/12¾oz skinless chicken breast,
   cut into strips

2 tbsp mayonnaise

1 garlic clove, crushed

1 tsp lemon juice

½ tsp stevia powder

2 anchovy fillets, drained and finely
   chopped

2 tbsp freshly grated Parmesan
   cheese

freshly ground black pepper

romaine lettuce, torn into pieces

Spicy Chicken Caesar Salad

Serves: 2

Preparation time:
20 minutes, plus
20 minutes marinating

Cooking time:
30 minutes

This is my own take on the traditional Caesar salad, with a little spicy kick to get the metabolism going at full speed.

1 Preheat the oven to 160°C/325°F/gas 3. Put the red pepper and tomatoes in an ovenproof dish and drizzle over the balsamic vinegar. Roast for 30 minutes.

2 Meanwhile, put the stock in a bowl with the chilli powder, crushed chilli flakes and coriander. Add the chicken strips and mix until well coated. Cover with cling film and leave to marinate at room temperature for about 20 minutes.

3 Mix together the mayonnaise, garlic, lemon juice, stevia powder, anchovies and Parmesan and season to taste with pepper. A little hot water can be added to thin the dressing if it is a little thick for your taste.

4 Put the chicken and marinade mixture in a non-stick saucepan over a medium heat and cook for about 10 minutes, stirring occasionally, until the chicken is cooked through and most of the liquid has evaporated. Top the lettuce with the chicken, tomatoes and red peppers, then drizzle over the dressing to serve.

NUTRITION NOTES
PER SERVING
• • • • • • • • • • • • • • • •
• Calories: 365kcals
• Fat: 18g
• Carbohydrates: 12g

2 garlic cloves, crushed

3 shallots, finely chopped

300g/10½oz minced turkey

1 tbsp balsamic vinegar

1 tsp chilli powder

1 tsp crushed dried red chilli flakes

2 tsp ground coriander

1 tsp stevia powder

½ vegetable stock cube, crumbled

1 tbsp soy sauce

1 egg white

2 large handfuls of mixed salad leaves, to serve

FOR THE SATAY SAUCE

2 tbsp peanut butter (no added sugar)

1 tsp ground ginger

1 tsp stevia powder

juice of ½ lime

90ml/3fl oz/generous ⅓ cup coconut milk

freshly ground black pepper

Turkey Kebabs with Satay Sauce

Serves: 2

Preparation time:
25 minutes, plus
1 hour chilling

Cooking time:
16 minutes

This sauce is so useful as it works well with just about any meat, but is especially good with turkey. And why save turkey for Christmas when it is one of the best meat choices to eat for good health?

1 Put the garlic and shallots in a non-stick saucepan over a low heat and cook for a few minutes to soften, adding a drop of water if it starts to stick. Remove from the heat and leave to cool slightly.

2 Put the mince, balsamic vinegar, chilli powder, crushed chilli flakes, coriander, stevia powder, stock cube and soy sauce in a large mixing bowl. Add the cooled shallots and garlic, then stir in the egg white. Using wet hands to stop the mixture sticking to you, mix all the ingredients together well. Cover with cling film and chill in the fridge for 1 hour. While the meat is in the fridge, put some wooden skewers into water to soak.

3 To make the sauce, put all the ingredients in a non-stick saucepan over a low heat and cook for 5 minutes until the peanut butter has melted and combined, stirring frequently. Gradually add boiling water 1 tablespoon at a time until you have the required consistency for a dipping sauce.

NUTRITION NOTES PER SERVING
· · · · · · · · · · · · · · ·
· Calories: 474kcals
· Fat: 30g
· Carbohydrates: 13g

4 Preheat the grill to high. To create the kebabs, take a small handful of the meat mixture and pack it around a skewer, spreading it evenly along the skewer. Repeat with the remaining skewers. Grill the skewers for about 7 minutes, turning regularly, until cooked through and browned.

5 Pour the sauce over the kebabs and serve with a mixed leaf salad.

400g/14oz skinless turkey steaks

1 handful of button mushrooms, finely chopped

½ tbsp red wine vinegar

100ml/3½fl oz/generous ⅓ cup chicken stock

2 tbsp double cream

1 tbsp finely chopped basil leaves

35g/1¼oz blue cheese, such as Stilton or Dolcelatte

½ red onion, sliced

8 cherry tomatoes, halved

½ yellow pepper, deseeded and sliced

freshly ground black pepper

2 handfuls of baby spinach leaves, to serve

Turkey in Cheesy Mushroom & Basil Sauce with Roast Vegetables

Serves: 2

Preparation time: 20 minutes

Cooking time: 35 minutes

With its rich, strong taste, the blue cheese makes this sauce truly indulgent, and combines with the sweet roast vegetables to create a real treat.

1 Preheat the oven to 180°C/350°F/gas 4. Put the turkey steaks in a non-stick frying pan over a low heat and gently brown on each side, then remove them from the pan and leave to one side. Add the mushrooms, wine vinegar and stock to the pan, season to taste with pepper and bring to the boil over a medium heat. Turn down the heat to low and leave to simmer for 10 minutes until the liquid has reduced and thickened a little.

2 Remove from the heat and add the cream, basil and blue cheese, then stir until the cheese has melted. Return the turkey to the sauce, then spoon everything into an ovenproof dish, cover with a lid and bake for 20 minutes until the turkey is cooked through and tender.

3 Meanwhile, put the onion, tomatoes and yellow pepper in a baking tray, cover with kitchen foil and bake for 20 minutes along with the turkey.

4 Serve the hot turkey and vegetables with a handful of fresh spinach leaves.

NUTRITION NOTES
PER SERVING
• • • • • • • • • • • • • • • • •
• Calories: 403kcals
• Fat: 18g
• Carbohydrates: 17g

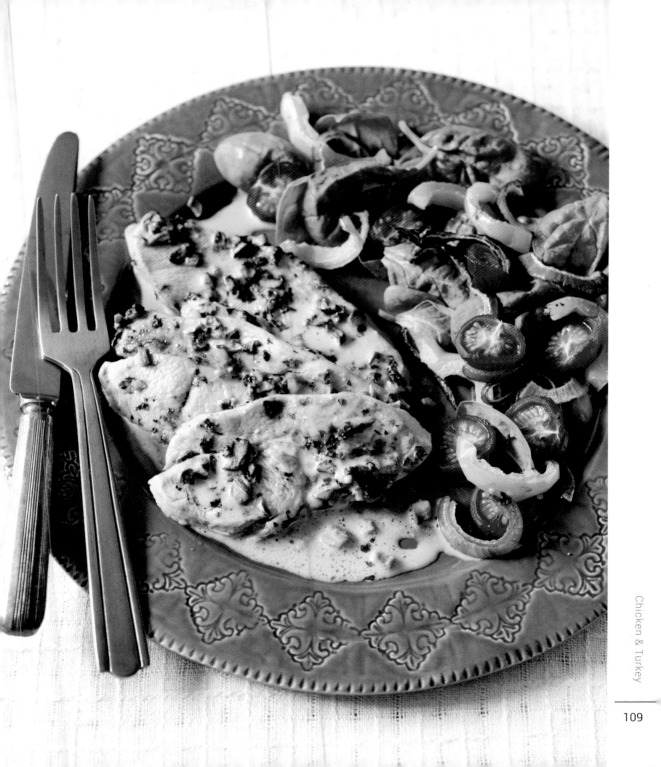

2 tbsp groundnut oil

4 garlic cloves, crushed

1 tsp grated root ginger

3 spring onions, chopped

½ small red cabbage, thinly sliced

½ red pepper, deseeded and sliced

10 sugar snap peas

200ml/7fl oz/scant 1 cup vegetable
   stock

1 tbsp soy sauce

1 tsp stevia powder

140g/5oz pork fillet, cut into thin
   strips

1 tbsp sesame seeds

Garlic Pork Stir-Fry

Serves: 2

Preparation time:
10 minutes

Cooking time:
15 minutes

This is primarily one for garlic-lovers, but don't discount it even if you don't count yourself among them – do give it a try. Garlic is an amazing ingredient that helps to fight infections and ward off colds as well as tasting great.

1 Heat a wok or large frying pan over a medium heat, then add the peanut oil, garlic, ginger and spring onions. Cook for a few minutes until the onions have softened.

2 Add the cabbage, red pepper, sugar snap peas, stock, soy sauce and stevia powder and stir together. Add the pork and continue to cook, uncovered, for about 5–10 minutes, stirring regularly, until the pork is tender.

3 Serve sprinkled with the sesame seeds.

NUTRITION NOTES
PER SERVING
• • • • • • • • • • • • • •
• Calories: 325kcals
• Fat: 19g
• Carbohydrates: 21g

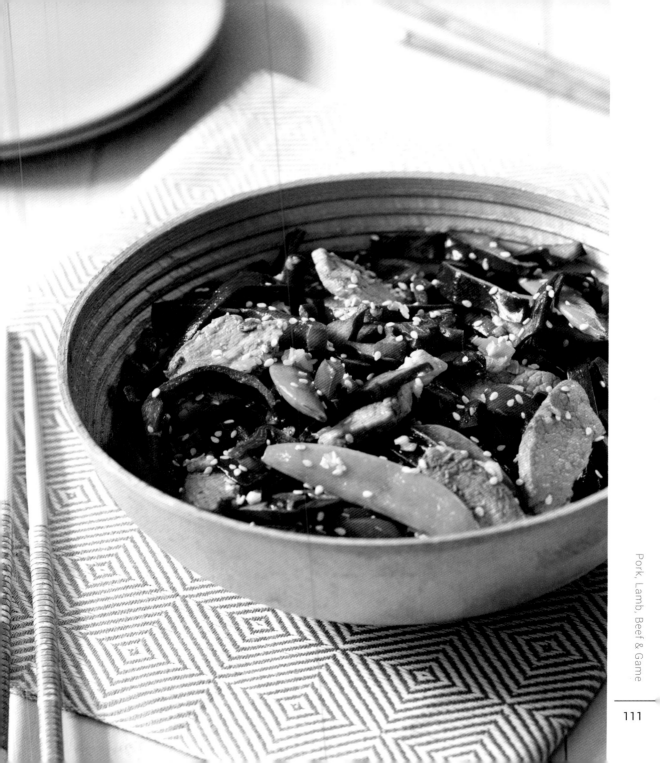

FOR THE EGG, PARMA HAM AND
   WALNUT SALAD

1 large handful of watercress

¼ red onion, finely chopped

2 large gherkins, finely chopped

1 celery stick, finely chopped

4 slices of Parma ham, cut into thin
   strips

2 eggs

a pinch of salt

FOR THE BLUE CHEESE DRESSING

2 tbsp mayonnaise

1 garlic clove, crushed

1 small handful of basil leaves,
   finely chopped

50g/1¾oz Stilton cheese, crumbled

freshly ground black pepper

Egg, Parma Ham & Walnut Salad with Blue Cheese Dressing

Serves: 2

Preparation time:
15 minutes

Cooking time:
5 minutes

Walnuts are highly nutritious so make a great addition to your everyday meals. They work perfectly alongside the strong flavours of this salad.

1   To make the salad, mix together the watercress, onion, gherkins and celery, then sprinkle the salad evenly with the Parma ham.

2   To make the dressing, mix together the mayonnaise, garlic and basil, crumble in the Stilton cheese and season to taste with pepper. Mix together well.

3   Bring a wide, shallow saucepan of lightly salted water to the boil over a high heat. Turn down the heat to low and stir the water vigorously. Break 1 egg into a cup, then slip it into the water. Repeat with the other egg. Simmer for 3–4 minutes until the whites have set but the yolks remain runny. Lift the poached eggs out of the water using a slotted spoon, put on top of the salad and drizzle with the blue cheese dressing to serve.

NUTRITION NOTES
PER SERVING
• • • • • • • • • • • • • • • •
• Calories: 355kcals
• Fat: 29g
• Carbohydrates: 3g

100ml/3½fl oz/generous ⅓ cup
  coconut milk
2 garlic cloves, crushed
1 tsp grated root ginger
1 tsp crushed dried red chilli flakes
1 tsp chilli powder
1 tsp turmeric
1 tsp ground coriander

1 tsp ground cumin
200ml/7fl oz/scant 1 cup fish stock
2 tbsp crunchy peanut butter
  (no added sugar)
1 tbsp fish sauce
½ tbsp stevia powder
½ tbsp lime juice
1 handful of broccoli florets

1 handful of mangetout
2 spring onions, chopped
140g/5oz minced pork
200g/7oz shirataki noodles, drained
  and rinsed
1 small handful of coriander leaves,
  chopped
freshly ground black pepper

Thai Pork Coco-Nutty Noodles

Serves: 2

Preparation time:
10 minutes

Cooking time:
20 minutes

A simple blend of Asian flavours, this noodle dish is really filling. I just love any kind of coconut-milk dish so it is one I make frequently.

1 Heat a wok or a heavy-based frying pan over a medium heat, add 1 tablespoon of the coconut milk with the garlic, ginger, crushed chilli flakes, chilli powder, turmeric, ground coriander, cumin, stock and peanut butter. Stir until the peanut butter has melted and the mixture combined. Add the fish sauce, stevia powder and lime juice and bring to the boil. Turn down the heat to low, add the vegetables and minced pork and cook for about 2 minutes, making sure you break up the mince well.

2 Add the remaining coconut milk and the noodles, return to the boil, then leave to simmer, uncovered, for a further 10 minutes.

3 Season to taste with pepper and serve sprinkled with the chopped coriander.

NUTRITION NOTES
PER SERVING
• • • • • • • • • • • • • • • •
• Calories: 417kcals
• Fat: 30g
• Carbohydrates: 13g

Pork, Lamb, Beef & Game

113

FOR THE CREAMY GARLIC DIP

1 spring onion, finely chopped

1 small red chilli, deseeded and
    chopped

4 garlic cloves, crushed

1 tsp grated root ginger

1 tsp chilli powder

2 tsp stevia powder

1 tbsp soy sauce

juice of 2 limes

2 tbsp cream cheese

300g/10½oz lamb fillet, cut into
    chunks

½ aubergine or 1 small aubergine,
    cut into chunks

1 tbsp vegetable oil

2 handfuls of rocket leaves

freshly ground black pepper

Lamb & Aubergine Kebabs with Creamy Garlic Dip

Serves: 2

Preparation time:
15 minutes

Cooking time:
20 minutes

These super-tender and succulent kebabs are served hot with the cold, fresh dip. The flavour of the dip is improved if you can prepare it the day before and chill it in the fridge overnight to allow the flavours to intensify.

1   Soak four wooden skewers in water. To make the dip, put the spring onion, red chilli and garlic in a heavy-based, non-stick saucepan and cook for a few minutes over a low heat until softened, adding a splash of water, if necessary, if the ingredients begin to stick. Add the ginger, chilli powder, stevia powder, soy sauce and lime juice and continue to cook for about 10 minutes, stirring regularly, until very soft and well blended. Remove from the heat and leave to cool slightly. Stir in the cream cheese and mix well.

2   Preheat the grill to high. Toss the lamb and aubergine in the oil until well coated, then season with pepper. Thread alternate pieces of lamb and aubergine on to the skewers and grill for about 10 minutes until cooked through, making sure your turn them regularly.

3   Serve the kebabs on a bed of rocket leaves with the garlic dip served separately.

NUTRITION NOTES
PER SERVING
• • • • • • • • • • • • • • • •
• **Calories: 316kcals**
• **Fat: 15g**
• **Carbohydrates: 11g**

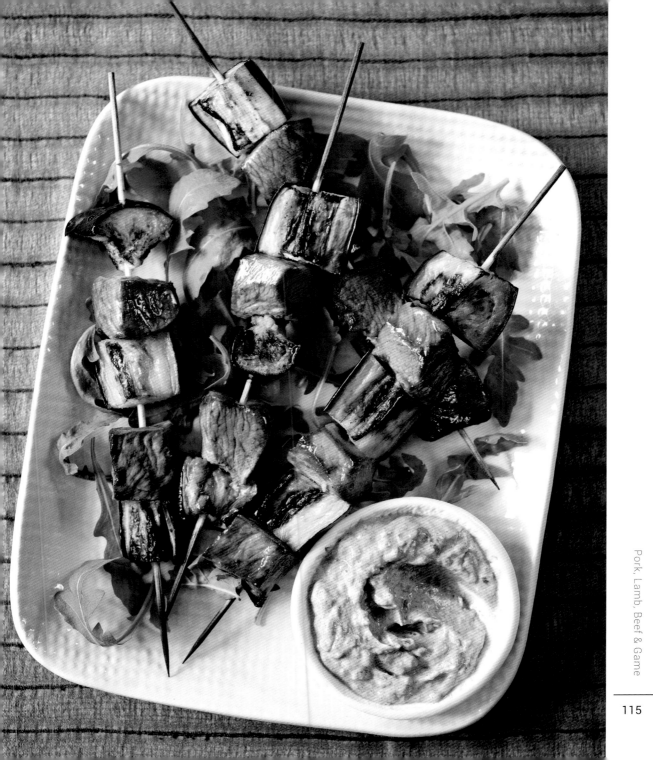

Pork, Lamb, Beef & Game

1 tbsp olive oil

½ red onion, finely chopped

1 celery stick, finely chopped

2 garlic cloves, crushed

300g/10½oz lamb fillet, cut into chunks

1 large leek, trimmed and chopped

2 carrots, diced

300ml/10½fl oz/scant 1¼ cups lamb stock

½ tbsp chopped rosemary leaves

1 tbsp mint sauce

1 tbsp tomato purée

1 tsp stevia powder

½ celeriac, peeled and chopped

½ small cauliflower, cut into florets

2 tbsp butter

freshly ground black pepper

Minty Lamb Casserole with Buttery Cauliflower & Celeriac Mash

Serves: 2

Preparation time: 20 minutes

Cooking time: 1 hour 40 minutes

This is a real hearty dish which I love to cook on a rainy Sunday afternoon. Its rich, thick gravy poured over the hot buttery mash makes for great comfort food.

1 Preheat the oven to 180°C/350°F/gas 4. Heat the oil in a heavy-based, flameproof casserole dish over a medium heat, add the onion, celery and garlic and cook for 5 minutes until soft. Add the lamb and fry for a few minutes until lightly browned. Add the leek, carrots, stock, rosemary, mint sauce, tomato purée and stevia powder. Bring to the boil, then cover with a lid and transfer to the oven for 1½ hours until the lamb is tender and the sauce has thickened.

2 After about 1 hour, put the celeriac into a saucepan of boiling water and return it to the boil. Turn down the heat to low, cover with a lid and leave to simmer for 10 minutes. Add the cauliflower florets and cook for a further 15 minutes until the vegetables are very soft. Drain well, then return to the pan, add the butter and season to taste with pepper. Mash together well and serve with the lamb.

NUTRITION NOTES
PER SERVING
• • • • • • • • • • • • • • • •
• Calories: 498kcals
• Fat: 29g
• Carbohydrates: 29g

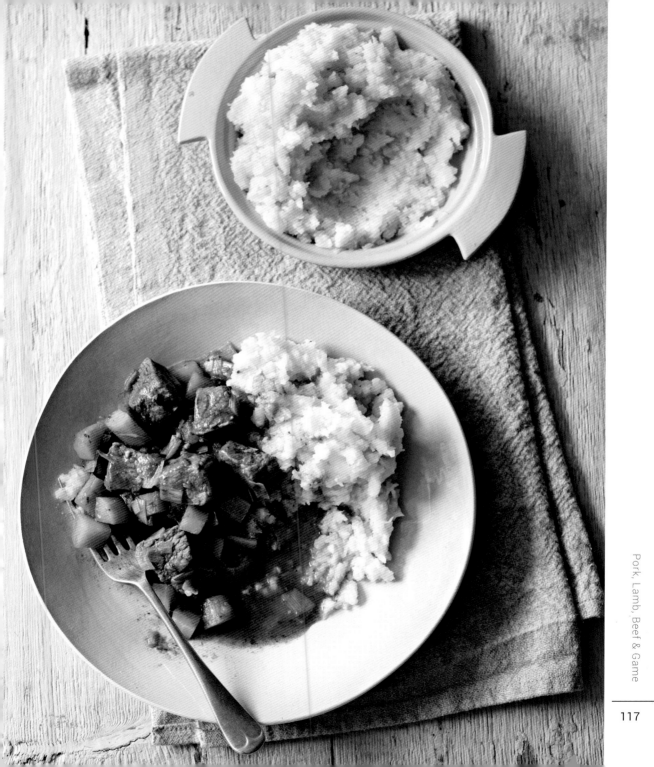

10 cherry tomatoes, chopped

15 black olives, pitted and sliced

1 red pepper, deseeded and diced

175g/6oz button mushrooms, sliced

2 tsp dried oregano

2 tbsp olive oil

½ tbsp red wine vinegar

2 lean beef steaks, each about
   100g/3½oz

2 garlic cloves, crushed

1 tsp stevia powder

200g/7oz cauliflower florets

freshly ground black pepper

Steak with Tomatoes & Olives

Serves: 2

Preparation time:
15 minutes

Cooking time:
30 minutes

This Mediterranean-inspired recipe works well with all meats and fish, so try it with lean lamb chops or a tender fish fillet instead of the steak. It is bursting with flavour and is so quick to make that it is ideal for a mid-week meal after work.

1   Put the tomatoes, olives, red pepper, mushrooms and oregano in a non-stick saucepan over a low heat and cook, uncovered, for about 10 minutes, stirring occasionally, until softened. Add the oil and wine vinegar and season to taste with pepper. Add the steaks and cook for a further 10–20 minutes, depending on how well you like your steak cooked.

2   Towards the end of the cooking time, cook the garlic, stevia powder and cauliflower florets in a separate saucepan over a low heat for 5–10 minutes, stirring regularly, until tender but not soggy.

3   Serve the steak and cauliflower with plenty of the tomato sauce.

NUTRITION NOTES
PER SERVING
• • • • • • • • • • • • • • • • •

• Calories: 297kcals
• Fat: 29g
• Carbohydrates: 11g

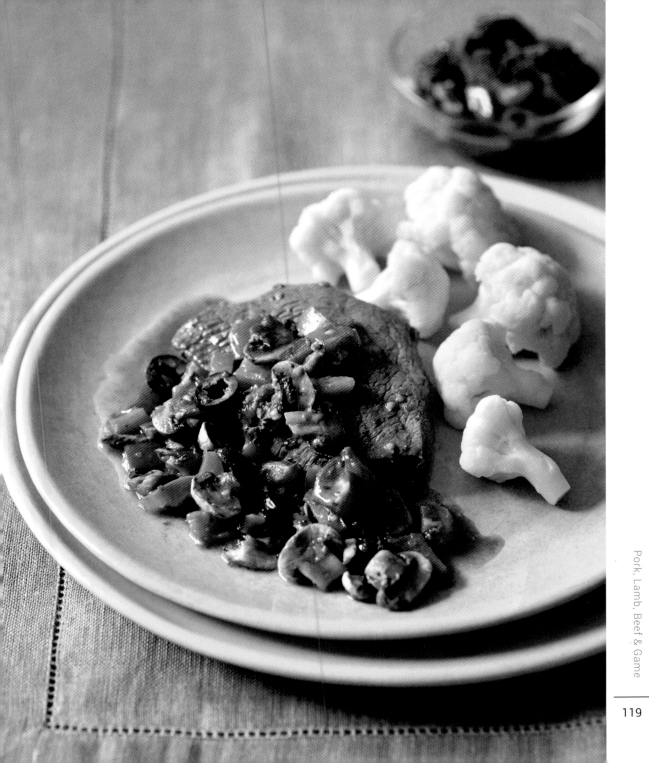

1 handful of coriander leaves, finely chopped

2 garlic cloves, crushed

1 tbsp crushed dried red chilli flakes

1 tsp stevia powder

½ tbsp fish sauce

juice of ½ lime

2 lean steaks, each about 100g/3½oz, cut into strips

40g/1½oz/¼ cup raw unsalted peanuts

1 tbsp vegetable oil

1 large carrot, cut into ribbons using a vegetable peeler

2 spring onions, finely chopped

½ red pepper, deseeded and finely chopped

1 shallot, finely chopped

8 little gem lettuce leaves

freshly ground black pepper

Spicy Thai Beef Little Gems

Serves: 2

Preparation time:
20 minutes, plus
1–2 hours marinating

Cooking time:
16 minutes

This delicious dish makes a lovely light evening meal, with its traditional Thai flavours of lime, chilli and fish sauce. They may be small but they are packed with flavour and goodness, and are surprisingly filling.

1 Reserve 1 tablespoon of chopped coriander, then mix the remainder with the garlic, crushed chilli flakes, stevia powder, fish sauce and lime juice in a non-metallic bowl. Blend the ingredients to a paste, using a hand-held blender. Add the steaks, cover with cling film and leave to marinate in the fridge for 1–2 hours.

2 Meanwhile, preheat the oven to 150°C/300°F/gas 2. Put the peanuts in a baking tray and roast for 10 minutes until golden. Remove from the oven and leave to cool slightly, then put into a bag or wrap in a kitchen towel and use a rolling pin to break them up into smaller pieces.

3 Heat the oil in a frying pan over a medium heat, add the carrot, spring onions, red pepper and shallot and cook for a few minutes until beginning to soften. Add the marinated steak with any remaining marinade and continue to cook for a further few minutes until the steak is cooked through.

4 Divide the mixture evenly between the little gem lettuce leaves. Sprinkle with the roasted nuts and the reserved coriander leaves and season to taste with pepper before serving.

NUTRITION NOTES
PER SERVING
• • • • • • • • • • • • • • • •
• Calories: 422kcals
• Fat: 38g
• Carbohydrates: 16g

1 tbsp olive oil

½ red onion, thinly sliced

½ red pepper, deseeded and thinly sliced

1 large carrot, cut into ribbons using a vegetable peeler

1 large handful of thinly shredded red cabbage

200g/7oz shirataki noodles, drained and rinsed

200g/7oz lean fillet steak, cut into thin strips

70ml/2¼fl oz/scant ⅓ cup beef stock

2 tbsp horseradish sauce

½ avocado, to serve

Beef & Horseradish Noodles

Serves: 2

Preparation time:
15 minutes

Cooking time:
15 minutes

This dish is super quick and easy. Shirataki noodles are always good for a speedy supper as they only need a quick rinse before reheating. If, like me, you love the kick of horseradish, then you will surely love this dish.

1   Heat the oil in a wok or heavy-based pan over a medium heat, add the onion and red pepper and cook for a few minutes. Add the carrot, cabbage and noodles and cook for a further 5 minutes, stirring occasionally.

2   Add the steak, stock and horseradish sauce, stir well and return to the boil. Turn down the heat to low and leave to simmer, uncovered, for a further 5 minutes.

3   Just before serving, peel, pit and slice the avocado. Serve the beef and noodles topped with the avocado slices.

NUTRITION NOTES
PER SERVING
•••••••••••••••••

• Calories: 414kcals
• Fat: 16g
• Carbohydrates: 14g

3 medium-thick slices of smoked
  bacon, rinded and chopped
1 tbsp butter
200g/7oz stewing steak, cut into
  small chunks
½ onion, finely chopped
1 garlic clove, crushed

1 bay leaf
1 tsp finely chopped thyme leaves
2 tsp finely chopped parsley leaves
500ml/17fl oz/2 cups chicken stock
1 carrot, diced
1 handful of button mushrooms,
  sliced

1 tbsp red wine vinegar
1 tsp stevia powder
1 tbsp tomato purée
200g/7oz cauliflower florets
freshly ground black pepper

Beef Bourguignon

Serves: 2

Preparation time:
20 minutes

Cooking time:
1¼ hours

Red meat shouldn't be eaten every day, as eating too much has been shown to put a strain on the kidneys and been strongly associated with increased risk of heart disease and other health problems. However, serving it once or twice a week is a really good way to get a boost of iron and B vitamins. This is a great recipe if you have a little time and freezes well if you want to make a large batch at the weekend.

1 Preheat the oven to 180°C/350°F/gas 4. Put the bacon and butter in a large, flameproof casserole dish over a medium heat and cook for about 5 minutes until the bacon is cooked through and slightly crisp. Add the steak and cook for a few minutes until the edges are sealed, then remove the beef and bacon from the pan.

2 Turn down the heat to low, add the onion and garlic to the pan with the bay leaf, thyme and parsley and cook for 5 minutes to soften. Return the beef and bacon to the pan with the stock, carrot, mushrooms, wine vinegar, stevia powder and tomato purée and season to taste with pepper. Increase the heat and bring to the boil, then cover with a lid and transfer to the oven for 1 hour until tender and well blended.

3 Meanwhile, put the cauliflower in a steamer, cover with a lid and steam for about 20 minutes until very soft. Once cooked, drain off any access water, then mash well, adding a little pepper to taste. Spoon the casserole straight from the dish and serve with the cauliflower mash.

NUTRITION NOTES
PER SERVING
• • • • • • • • • • • • • • • •
• Calories: 414kcals
• Fat: 17g
• Carbohydrates: 28g

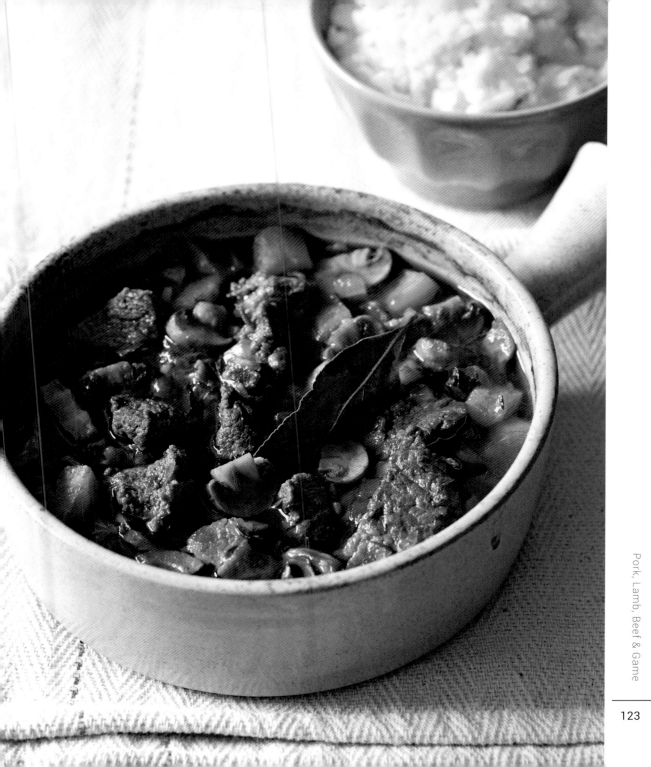

30g/1oz/scant ¼ cup walnuts

260g/9¼oz venison, sliced

100ml/3½fl oz/generous ⅓ cup
    beef stock

½ onion, finely chopped

1 carrot, finely chopped

1 large garlic clove, crushed

1 large handful of mushrooms, sliced

½ tbsp red wine vinegar

1 tbsp tomato purée

1 bay leaf

1 tsp finely chopped thyme leaves

½ tsp smoked paprika

2 large handfuls of kale

2 tbsp crème fraîche

freshly ground black pepper

Venison & Walnut Stroganoff with Steamed Kale

Serves: 2

Preparation time:
25 minutes

Cooking time:
20 minutes

A rich sauce perfectly sets off the lean and flavoursome venison. Teamed with healthy kale, you can't go wrong with this meal.

1   Put the walnuts into a saucepan of boiling water, return to the boil, then turn down the heat to low and leave to simmer for 5 minutes. Drain and leave until cool enough to handle, then chop finely.

2   Meanwhile, heat a large non-stick frying pan over a medium heat, add the sliced venison and cook for a few minutes until it starts to brown around the edges. Remove from the pan. Add a splash of the stock to the pan, then add the onion, carrot and garlic and cook for about 5 minutes. Add the remaining stock with the mushrooms, walnuts, wine vinegar, tomato purée, bay leaf, thyme and smoked paprika and season to taste with pepper. Bring to the boil, then turn down the heat to low, cover with a lid and leave to simmer for 20 minutes.

3   Put the kale in a steamer, cover with a lid and steam for 3 minutes until just tender but not soggy.

4   Return the venison to the sauce, stir in the crème fraîche and cook for a further 5 minutes, without allowing the mixture to boil. Serve the stroganoff on a bed of steamed kale.

NUTRITION NOTES
PER SERVING
● ● ● ● ● ● ● ● ● ● ● ● ● ● ●
• Calories: 634kcals
• Fat: 39g
• Carbohydrates: 18g

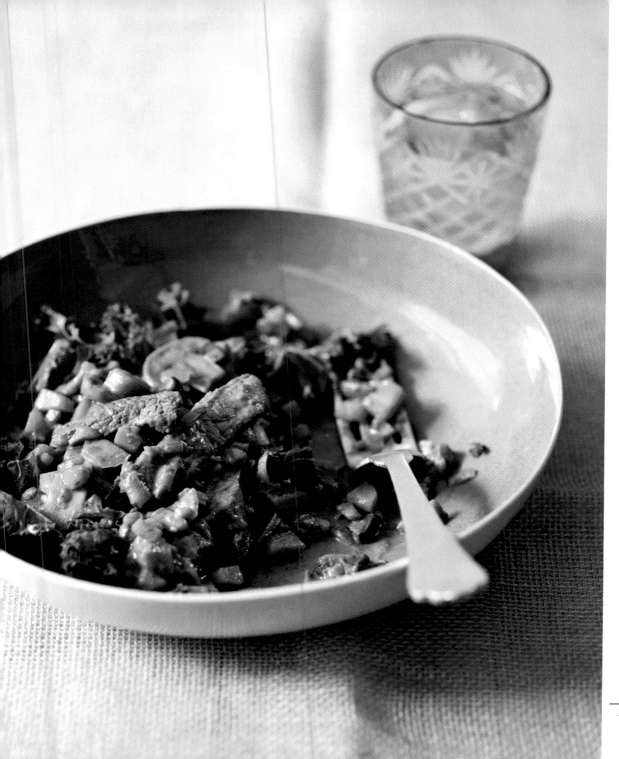

FOR THE SPICY VENISON

1 tsp ground cumin

1 tsp chilli powder

1 garlic clove, crushed

1 tsp finely chopped coriander leaves

1 tsp crushed dried red chilli flakes

1 tbsp soy sauce

1 tbsp Worcestershire sauce

1 tbsp olive oil

260g/9¼oz venison steak, cut into strips

FOR THE BLUE CHEESE SALAD

2 handfuls of baby spinach leaves

¼ cucumber, chopped

¼ red onion, sliced

50g/1¾oz blue cheese, diced

1 tbsp olive oil

juice of ½ lemon

1 tsp stevia powder

freshly ground black pepper

Spicy Venison with Blue Cheese Salad

Serves: 2

Preparation time:
20 minutes, plus
30 minutes marinating

Cooking time:
5 minutes

Venison has to be my favourite meat so it is always a bit of a treat for me. It's lean and delicious while being healthier than beef. Combined with the blue cheese, it makes a perfect partnership.

1   To make the spicy marinade, mix the cumin, chilli powder, garlic, coriander, crushed chilli flakes, soy sauce, Worcestershire sauce and olive oil in a bowl and mix well. Add the venison strips, cover with cling film and leave to marinate in the fridge for at least 30 minutes.

2   Put the spinach, cucumber, onion and cheese in a large salad bowl. In a separate bowl, whisk the olive oil with the lemon juice and stevia powder, then season to taste with pepper. Pour the dressing over the salad and toss to coat the leaves.

3   Heat a non-stick frying pan over a medium heat, add the venison and the marinade and cook for about 3–5 minutes, or until the venison is cooked to your liking. Serve the salad topped with the strips of venison with the dressing drizzled over.

NUTRITION NOTES
PER SERVING
● ● ● ● ● ● ● ● ● ● ● ● ● ● ●
• Calories: 452kcals
• Fat: 25g
• Carbohydrates: 10g

2½ tbsp double cream

½ large avocado, peeled, pitted and chopped

400g/14oz cooked or tinned white crab meat

2 tsp lemon juice

1 spring onion, finely chopped

2 handfuls of rocket leaves

2 handfuls of watercress

a sprinkle of paprika

freshly ground black pepper

Avocado Crab Salad

Serves: 2

Preparation time:
15 minutes, plus
30 minutes chilling

Super quick and easy, this luxurious dish makes a delicious treat and is especially good during the summer. If you use tinned crab meat, it really keeps the cost down but the dish still tastes amazing. Pile your plate with plenty of fresh salad, then top with the moulded crab salad.

1 Line two small cups or ramekins with cling film. In a large bowl, whisk the cream until frothy. Add the avocado, crab meat, lemon juice and spring onion, mix together well and season to taste with pepper. Divide the mixture between the prepared cups and press it down gently but firmly. Fold the cling film over the top to cover and seal, then chill in the fridge for 30 minutes.

2 Turn the pressed salad on to plates of rocket and watercress and sprinkle with paprika to serve.

**NUTRITION NOTES
PER SERVING**
• • • • • • • • • • • • • • • • •
• Calories: 224kcals
• Fat: 12g
• Carbohydrates: 6g

260g/9¼oz skinless salmon fillet, cut into chunks

2 eggs

3 tbsp double cream

1 tsp lemon juice

1 tbsp chopped dill leaves

½ tsp cayenne pepper

low-calorie cooking oil spray

2 handfuls of rocket leaves

freshly ground black pepper

FOR THE TOMATO AND RED PEPPER SALSA

½ red onion, finely chopped

½ red pepper, deseeded and finely chopped

3 large tomatoes, finely chopped

1 tbsp chopped coriander leaves

1 garlic clove, crushed

juice of ½ lime

1 tsp stevia powder

Salmon Terrine with Tomato & Red Pepper Salsa

Serves: 2

Preparation time: 20 minutes, plus 2 hours chilling

Cooking time: 30 minutes

I love making this dish. It is always such a hit because it looks so elegant and special. Leave it to chill for a few hours before serving, if you can, to allow the delicate flavours to meld together.

1   Preheat the oven to 180°C/350°F/gas 4. In a large bowl, mix together the salmon, eggs, cream, lemon juice, dill and cayenne, then season to taste with pepper. Blend the ingredients together to a smooth paste, using a hand-held blender.

2   Spray a 450g/1lb non-stick loaf tin with the low-calorie oil spray, then add the mixture to the tin. Put this tin into a larger, deeper baking tray and fill the outer tin with boiling water to come about halfway up the sides of the loaf tin. Bake for about 30 minutes. Leave to cool in the tin, then cover with cling film and chill in the fridge for a few hours before serving.

3   Mix together all the salsa ingredients, and season to taste with pepper. Turn out and slice the terrine, put on top of the rocket and dot with a spoonful of the salsa.

NUTRITION NOTES
PER SERVING
• • • • • • • • • • • • • • • •
• Calories: 361kcals
• Fat: 15g
• Carbohydrates: 6g

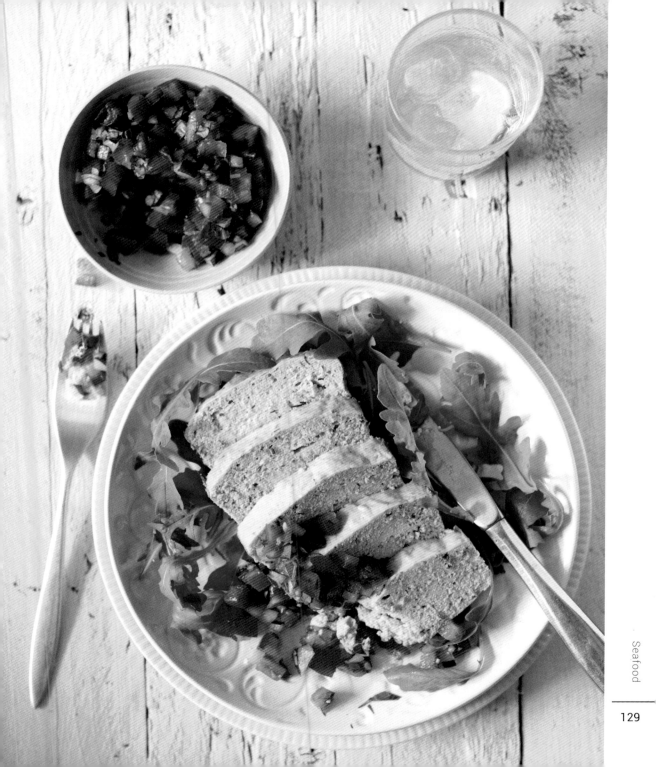

40 black olives, pitted

1 garlic clove, crushed

2 tbsp chopped coriander leaves

1 tbsp olive oil

4 sun-dried tomatoes

1 tsp lemon juice

12 asparagus spears, trimmed

2 salmon steaks, each about
125g/4½oz

freshly ground black pepper

Mediterranean Salmon with Asparagus

Serves: 2

Preparation time:
15 minutes

Cooking time:
20 minutes

Salmon should be eaten as often as possible on this diet plan and this recipe combines tender salmon with lots of fantastic Mediterranean flavours to give you that sunny summer-holiday feeling.

1   Preheat the oven to 220°C/425°F/gas 7. Put the olives, garlic, coriander, olive oil, sun-dried tomatoes and lemon juice in a non-metallic bowl and season with pepper. Blend the ingredients to a smooth paste, using a hand-held blender.

2   Put the asparagus on a sheet of kitchen foil and sprinkle with pepper. Bring the foil up over the asparagus, sealing the edges to form an airtight parcel. Bake for about 15–20 minutes.

3   Meanwhile, put the salmon steaks on to a sheet of kitchen foil and spread the paste evenly over the top. Seal the kitchen foil around the salmon to make an airtight parcel and put it on a baking tray. Bake for about 5 minutes.

4   Open up the salmon parcel, exposing the paste topping, and return the fish to the oven for a further 5 minutes, or until the salmon is cooked through. Unwrap both parcels and serve the olive salmon with the tender asparagus.

NUTRITION NOTES
PER SERVING
••••••••••••••••
• Calories: 365kcals
• Fat: 22g
• Carbohydrates: 7g

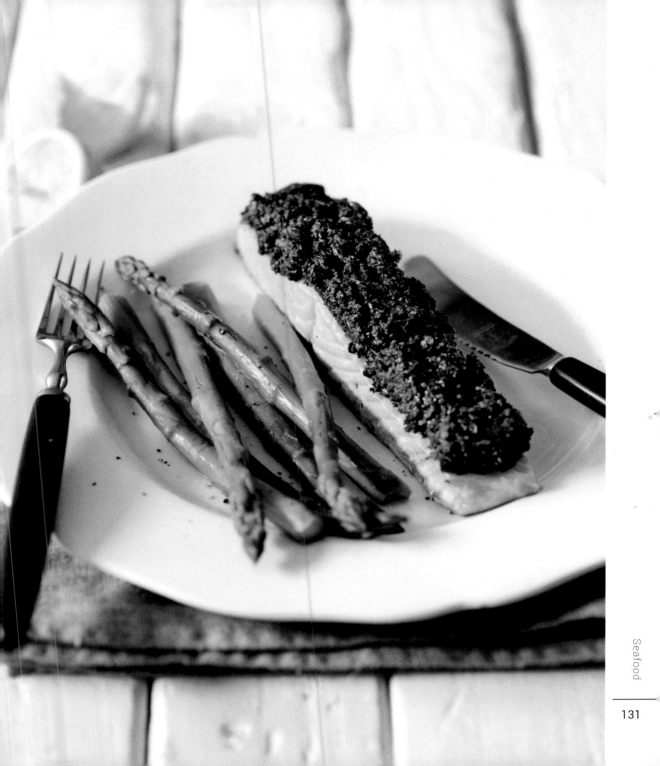

¼ large cauliflower, cut into florets

¼ red onion, finely chopped

¼ red pepper, deseeded and finely chopped

1 garlic clove, crushed

400g/14oz skinless undyed smoked cod, cut into chunks

1 egg white

55g/2oz Cheddar cheese, grated

a pinch of smoked paprika

2 handfuls of watercress

freshly ground black pepper

FOR THE DILL AND SPRING ONION MAYONNAISE

1 tbsp finely chopped dill leaves

1 tsp lemon juice

1 spring onion, finely chopped

2 tbsp mayonnaise

Smoked Cod Fishcakes with Dill & Spring Onion Mayonnaise

Serves: 2

Preparation time: 25 minutes, plus 10 minutes cooling and 1 hour chilling

Cooking time: 30 minutes

These low-carb fishcakes are really delicious and crisp on the outside but soft and tender in the middle. Use salmon instead of cod if you prefer.

1   Put the cauliflower florets in a steamer and steam for about 15 minutes until just soft. Drain and mash, then leave to cool.

2   While they are cooling, heat a non-stick saucepan over a low heat, add the onion, red pepper and garlic and cook for about 5 minutes until softened. Add the cod and cook for a further 5 minutes until the cod is starting to flake. Remove from the heat, drain off any liquid, then transfer to a bowl and leave to cool slightly.

3   Add the cauliflower mash, the egg white, Cheddar and paprika to the cod mixture, then season to taste with pepper. Mix the ingredients together well, then cover with cling film and chill in the fridge for 1 hour.

4   Preheat the grill to medium and line the grill pan with kitchen foil. Using wet hands to stop the mixture sticking to you, shape the mixture into 4 quite soft patties, then grill for about 4 minutes on each side until slightly golden.

5   Meanwhile, gently stir the dill, lemon juice and spring onion into the mayonnaise. Serve the hot fishcakes with a handful of watercress and a large dollop of the dill and onion mayonnaise.

NUTRITION NOTES
PER SERVING
• • • • • • • • • • • • • • • • •
• Calories: 482kcals
• Fat: 11g
• Carbohydrates: 12g

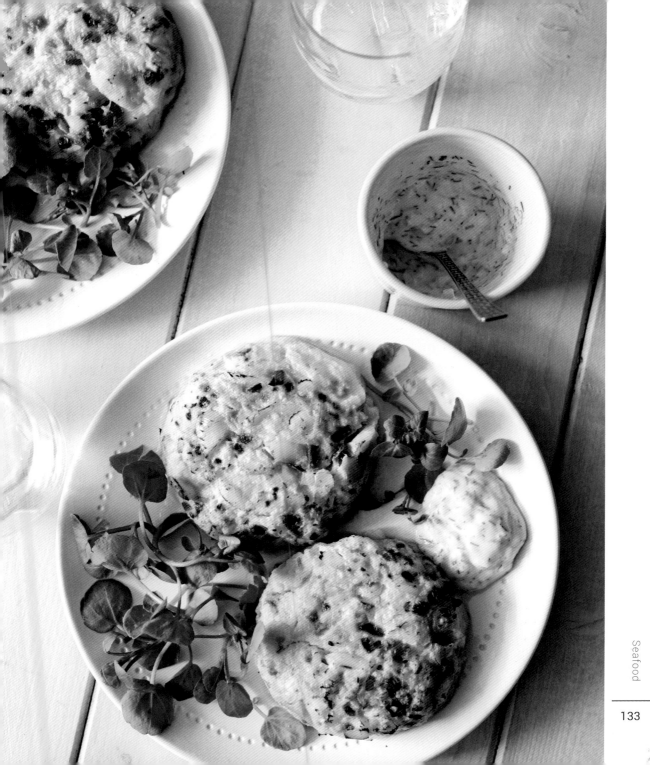

2 tbsp olive oil

½ onion, finely chopped

1 large carrot, finely chopped

½ red pepper, deseeded and finely chopped

1 garlic clove, crushed

1 tsp ground cumin

1 tsp crushed dried red chilli flakes

½ tsp ground cinnamon

a pinch of cayenne pepper

250ml/9fl oz/1 cup fish stock

400g/14oz tinned chopped plum tomatoes

1 tbsp tomato purée

juice of ½ lemon

20 green olives, pitted

1 tsp stevia powder

½ tsp smoked paprika

400g/14oz skinless cod fillet, cut into chunks

1 handful of coriander leaves, chopped

freshly ground black pepper

Spicy Moroccan Fish Stew

Serves: 2

Preparation time:
15 minutes

Cooking time:
30 minutes

This wonderfully exotic dish will really warm you through and get your circulation moving. The tender fish, flavoured with delicate spices, is sure to become one that the whole family will enjoy.

1   Put the oil, onion, carrot, red pepper, garlic, cumin, crushed chilli flakes, cinnamon and cayenne in a large, heavy-based saucepan over a medium heat, season to taste with pepper and cook for about 5 minutes, stirring regularly. Add the stock, tomatoes, tomato purée, lemon juice and olives and bring to the boil. Turn down the heat to low and leave to simmer, uncovered, for 10 minutes.

2   Add the stevia powder, paprika and cod and cook for a further 5–10 minutes until the fish flakes easily and the sauce is well blended. Serve the cod sprinkled with the chopped coriander.

NUTRITION NOTES
PER SERVING
• • • • • • • • • • • • • • • • •
• Calories: 477kcals
• Fat: 21g
• Carbohydrates: 24g

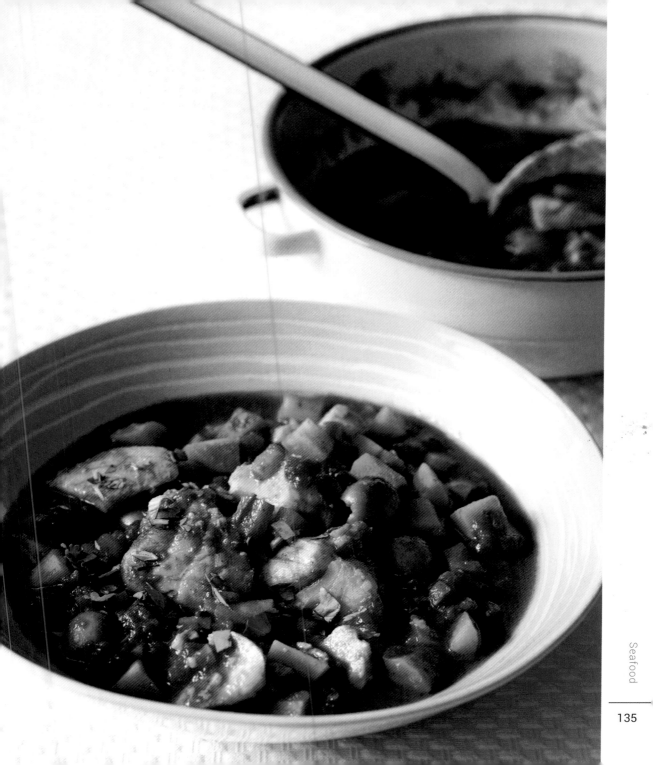

40g/1½oz/¼ cup raw unsalted
    peanuts
1 egg white
a pinch of cayenne pepper
a pinch of hot chilli powder
a pinch of turmeric

2 skinless haddock fillets, each about
    200g/7oz
2 handfuls of rocket leaves
½ cucumber, cut into ribbons using
    a vegetable peeler
1 spring onion, finely sliced

2 tbsp olive oil
1 tbsp balsamic vinegar
freshly ground black pepper
½ lime, sliced, to serve

Haddock with Spiced Cayenne Peanuts

Serves: 2

Preparation time:
15 minutes

Cooking time:
12 minutes

I always prefer the taste of haddock to cod, and combined with nuts in this dish it makes a heart-healthy, nutritious meal, full of goodness and flavour, and beautifully colourful, too (see pages 96–97).

1   Preheat the oven to 180°C/350°F/gas 4 and line a baking tray with baking paper. Mix together the peanuts, egg white, cayenne, chilli powder and turmeric in a bowl. Spread the mixture on to the prepared baking tray and bake for 5 minutes until crisp. Leave to cool slightly, then break into small pieces.

2   Preheat the grill to medium. Grill the haddock for a few minutes on each side until the fish flakes easily when tested with a fork.

3   Meanwhile, mix together the rocket, cucumber and spring onion. Whisk together the olive oil and balsamic vinegar in a small bowl, then season with a little pepper. Drizzle the dressing over the salad and toss gently, then top with the fish, sprinkle with the coated peanuts and serve with a slice of lime.

NUTRITION NOTES
PER SERVING
• • • • • • • • • • • • • • • •
• Calories: 363kcals
• Fat: 25g
• Carbohydrates: 12g

8 cherry tomatoes, halved

20 green olives, pitted and sliced

2 small handfuls of diced aubergine

2 garlic cloves, crushed

juice of 1 lemon

2 tbsp olive oil

6 basil leaves, finely chopped

400g/14oz firm tofu, diced

200g/7oz small broccoli florets

freshly ground black pepper

Tender Tomato & Olive Tofu

Serves: 2

Preparation time:
15 minutes, plus
1 hour marinating

Cooking time:
25 minutes

If you usually find tofu rather bland – and many people do – put aside that thought and give this recipe a try. The tofu really absorbs the strong flavours of the other ingredients – plus it makes a pleasant change from meat and fish.

1 Mix together the cherry tomatoes, olives, aubergine, garlic, lemon juice, olive oil and basil in a non-metallic bowl, then season to taste with pepper. Add the tofu, cover with cling film and leave to marinate in the fridge for 1 hour.

2 Heat a non-stick frying pan over a medium-low heat, add the tofu mixture and bring to the boil. Turn down the heat to low, cover with a lid and leave to simmer for about 20 minutes until the aubergine is soft.

3 Towards the end of the cooking time, put the broccoli florets in a steamer, cover with a lid and steam for a few minutes until tender. Serve the tofu on a bed of steamed broccoli.

NUTRITION NOTES
PER SERVING
● ● ● ● ● ● ● ● ● ● ● ● ● ● ● ● ●
• Calories: 357kcals
• Fat: 22g
• Carbohydrates: 17g

Seafood / Vegetarian

137

½ red chilli, deseeded and finely
   chopped
1 garlic clove, crushed
1 large handful of coriander leaves,
   chopped

30g/1oz/heaped ¼ cup cashew nuts
3 tbsp sesame oil
1 tsp lime juice
300g/10½oz firm tofu, cut into thick
   strips

1 large handful of mangetout
200g/7oz shirataki noodles, drained
   and rinsed
freshly ground black pepper

Asian-Style Pesto & Tofu Noodles

Serves: 2

Preparation time:
10 minutes

Cooking time:
8 minutes

Asian pesto has a great kick to it and tastes deliciously fresh. Drizzled over this vegetarian staple and served with the noodles really makes for a quick but flavoursome and highly satisfying meal.

1   To make the pesto, put the chilli, garlic, coriander, cashews, 2 tablespoons of the sesame oil and the lime juice in a non-metallic bowl, then season to taste with pepper. Blend the ingredients together well, using a hand-held blender.

2   Heat the remaining sesame oil in a non-stick frying pan over a medium heat, add the tofu and cook for a few minutes, tossing gently, until the tofu is just beginning to turn golden.

3   Add the mangetout and noodles and cook over a medium heat for about 4 minutes, stirring regularly. Stir the pesto through the other ingredients and serve hot.

NUTRITION NOTES
PER SERVING
• • • • • • • • • • • • • • • •
• Calories: 393kcals
• Fat: 30g
• Carbohydrates: 9g

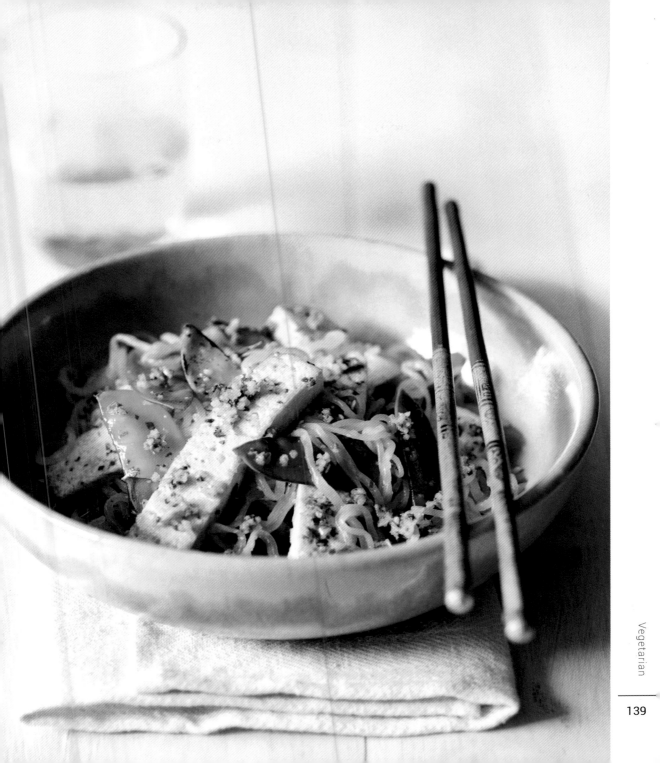

2 large mushrooms, stems removed

2 shallots, finely chopped

1 garlic clove, crushed

4 chive stalks, finely chopped

60g/2¼oz mozzarella cheese, grated

freshly ground black pepper

**FOR THE BROCCOLI AND
SUNFLOWER SEED SALAD**

¼ red onion, finely chopped

¼ red pepper, deseeded and finely
chopped

1 tbsp balsamic vinegar

2 tsp agave nectar

2 handfuls of small broccoli florets

2 tbsp sunflower seeds

2 tbsp mayonnaise

1 tsp apple cider vinegar

Stuffed Mushrooms with Broccoli & Sunflower Seed Salad

Serves: 2

Preparation time:
15 minutes

Cooking time:
20 minutes

This is a lovely, light vegetarian meal and a great source of protein and calcium. The broccoli salad is surprisingly yummy.

1   Preheat the oven to180°C/350°F/gas 4. Put the mushroom caps, gill-side up, on a baking tray. Mix together the shallots, garlic, chives and mozzarella, then season to taste with pepper. Spoon the mixture into the mushrooms and pat down, then bake for about 20 minutes until golden.

2   Meanwhile, put the onion, red pepper, balsamic vinegar and 1 teaspoon of the agave nectar in a non-stick saucepan over a medium heat and cook, uncovered, for a few minutes until softened slightly. Add the broccoli and sunflower seeds and cook for a further 1 minute to warm through. Leave to cool slightly. Mix together the mayonnaise, cider vinegar and the remaining agave nectar, then stir into the broccoli mixture.

3   Serve the baked mushrooms hot with the broccoli salad.

**NUTRITION NOTES
PER SERVING**
• • • • • • • • • • • • • • • •
• Calories: 284kcals
• Fat: 20g
• Carbohydrates: 16g

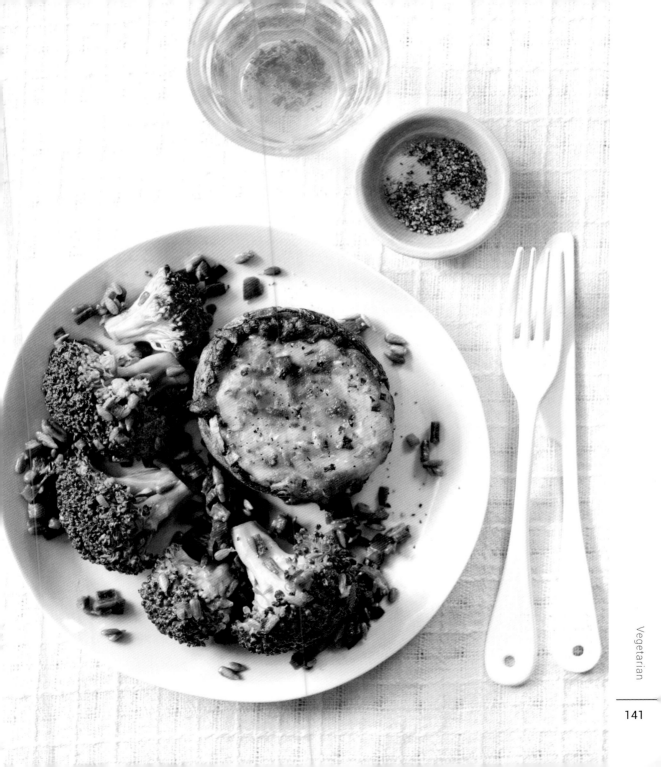

CHAPTER 5
DESSERT RECIPES

Now to my favourite section … desserts! Most people assume they can no longer enjoy desserts on a diet and, to be honest, for optimum weight loss they are better avoided. But a diet plan is about learning to eat healthily to maintain an optimum weight, and to do that we need to be able to incorporate treats into our lives without feeling guilty or piling on the pounds. But don't get too excited as these desserts – like this Almond Apple Crumble (see page 151) – come with one important rule: you can only have one once a week, so you need to think of your dessert as a weekend treat. But the added bonus is that getting a larger hit of calories once a week prevents your body from getting used to a set number of calories and stranding you on a weight-loss plateau.

These desserts do contain carbohydrate, but they have been prepared with a good level of fat and protein to ensure that you don't get a massive rise in blood sugar levels. So take your time with your dessert and really enjoy your weekly treat … you deserve it!

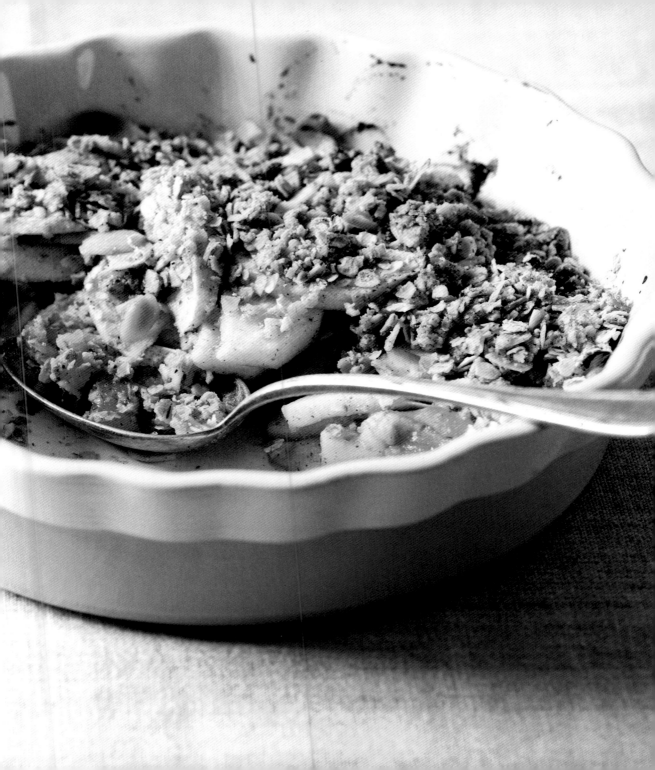

30g/1oz/scant ¼ cup raw unsalted
   peanuts
50g/1¾oz dark chocolate, 70% cocoa
   solids, broken into pieces
10 large strawberries, hulled

Nutty Chocolate-Covered Strawberries

Serves: 2

Preparation time:
15 minutes, plus
30 minutes chilling

Cooking time:
20 minutes

These may be super simple to prepare but they are always a huge hit with my friends. Just by adding the nuts to a basic recipe, you create a real taste sensation. Another option for your melted chocolate is to pour it over chunks of banana, hot from baking in their skins in a moderate oven for 15 minutes, then sprinkle them with chopped hazelnuts to serve.

1   Preheat the oven to 180°C/350°F/gas 4. Put the peanuts on a baking tray and bake for 20 minutes until golden.

2   Meanwhile, put the chocolate in a large heatproof bowl and rest it over a pan of gently simmering water, making sure that the bottom of the bowl does not touch the water. Heat, stirring occasionally, until the chocolate has melted. Remove the bowl from the heat.

3   Remove the peanuts from the oven and leave to cool slightly, then chop finely and put on a plate.

4   Take 1 strawberry at a time, press a thin skewer into the centre so that you can roll it first into the melted chocolate to coat, then in the peanuts, then put them on a plate. When they are all coated, chill them in the fridge for at least 30 minutes before serving.

NUTRITION NOTES
PER SERVING
••••••••••••••••••
• Calories: 188kcals
• Fat: 14g
• Carbohydrates: 13g

1 pear, peeled, halved and cored

1 tbsp butter

1 tsp stevia powder

1 tsp ground cinnamon

1½ tbsp natural yogurt

1 passionfruit, halved and seeds scooped out

1 tbsp agave nectar

4 mint leaves

Pear Passion with Agave Yogurt

Serves: 2

Preparation time:
10 minutes

Cooking time:
20 minutes

This is another really simple dish that is fresh and healthy and full of vitamins and minerals. Serve it hot straight from the oven with a dollop of cold yogurt spooned over the top.

1 Preheat the oven to 180°C/350°F/gas 4. Put the pear halves, cut-sides up, in a baking tray and dot each half with the butter. Sprinkle over the stevia powder and cinnamon, then bake for 20 minutes until the pears are tender.

2 Put the yogurt, passionfruit seeds and agave nectar in a bowl and mix together.

3 Spoon the yogurt over the baked pears and top with the mint leaves to serve.

NUTRITION NOTES
PER SERVING
● ● ● ● ● ● ● ● ● ● ● ● ● ● ● ●
• Calories: 121kcals
• Fat: 7g
• Carbohydrates: 14g

Simple Desserts

½ tbsp butter

2 tsp agave nectar

10 pecan nuts

40g/1½oz dark chocolate, 70% cocoa
solids, broken into pieces

1½ tbsp natural yogurt

1 tsp finely grated lime zest

½ tsp hot chilli powder

2 egg whites

Chilli Lime Chocolate Mousse with Candied Pecans

Serves: 2

Preparation time:
10 minutes, plus
1 hour chilling

Cooking time:
10 minutes

You'll just love this real chocolate fix. And if you haven't tasted chocolate with chilli and lime, you really must give it a try – you will be amazed at how good it is.

1   Preheat the oven to 180°C/350°C/gas 4 and line a baking tray with baking paper.

2   Put the butter and 1 teaspoon of the agave nectar in a saucepan over a low heat until melted. Add the pecans and mix together well, then spread over the prepared baking tray. Bake for 10 minutes, then remove from the oven and leave to one side.

3   Meanwhile, put the chocolate in a large heatproof bowl and rest it over a pan of gently simmering water, making sure that the bottom of the bowl does not touch the water. Heat, stirring occasionally, until the chocolate has melted. Remove from the heat and stir for a moment until beginning to cool, then stir in the yogurt, lime zest and chilli powder.

4   In a separate bowl, whisk the egg whites and the remaining agave nectar until they form stiff peaks. Fold 1 tablespoon of the egg whites into the chocolate to loosen it, then carefully fold in the remainder, keeping as much air in the mixture as possible. Spoon into two ramekins or dessert glasses, then chill in the fridge for at least 1 hour. Sprinkle with the candied pecans to serve.

NUTRITION NOTES
PER SERVING
• • • • • • • • • • • • • • • •
• Calories: 279kcals
• Fat: 23g
• Carbohydrates: 11g

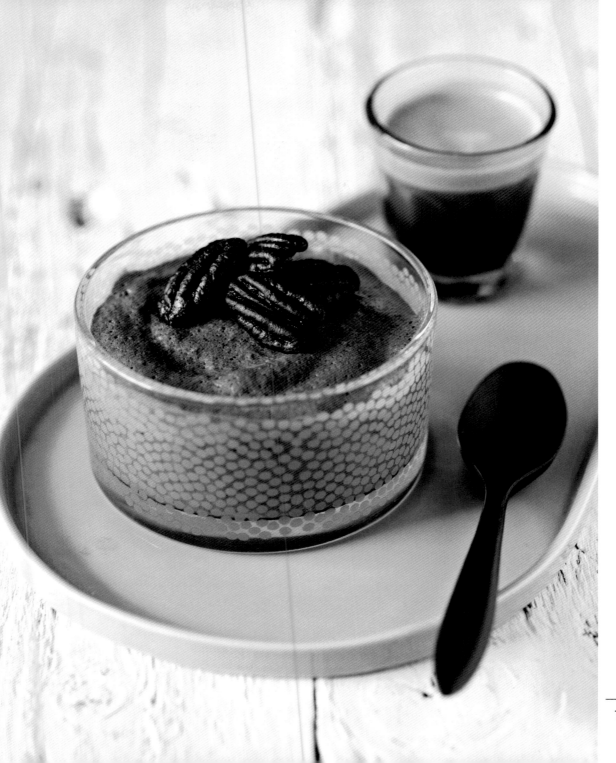

1 tbsp butter

1 tsp ground cinnamon

½ tbsp agave nectar

1 heaped tbsp whole almonds, roughly chopped

35g/1¼oz/⅓ cup rolled oats

1 handful of raspberries

1 tsp instant coffee granules, or more to taste

1 tbsp warm milk

2 tbsp ricotta cheese

1 tsp vanilla extract

25g/1oz dark chocolate, 70% cocoa solids, grated

Raspberry Mocha Tiramisu

Serves: 2

Preparation time:
15 minutes, plus
10 minutes cooling

Cooking time:
25 minutes

This has to be my favourite dessert recipe as I just love the combination of coffee and chocolate. Served at a dinner party, these beautifully presented desserts look really impressive.

1   Preheat the oven to 170°C/325°F/gas 3 and line a baking tray with baking paper.

2   Melt the butter in a non-stick saucepan over a low heat, add the cinnamon and agave nectar and cook for 1 minute until the the ingredients have combined. Remove from the heat. Stir in the almonds and oats, then spread the mixture evenly over the prepared baking tray. Bake for 20 minutes, then remove from the oven and leave to cool on the tray.

3   Divide the mixture between two large wine or dessert glasses and press down gently to make it firm. Squash the raspberries slightly with a fork, then put them on top of the oat base.

4   In a bowl, mix the coffee granules into the warm milk, adding a little more coffee if you prefer a stronger flavour. Stir until the granules have dissolved, then leave to cool. Stir in the ricotta and vanilla extract, then beat together well to form a smooth, creamy consistency. Spoon the mixture equally into the glasses and sprinkle with the grated chocolate.

NUTRITION NOTES
PER SERVING
• • • • • • • • • • • • • • • • •
• Calories: 380kcals
• Fat: 29g
• Carbohydrates: 20g

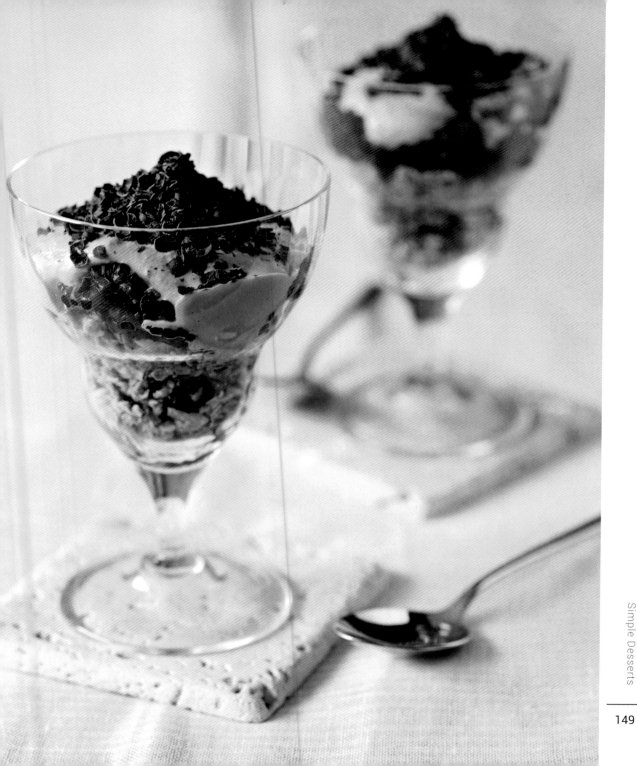

2 sheets of filo pastry

low-calorie cooking oil spray

150g/5½oz ricotta cheese

1 tsp vanilla extract

2 tsp stevia powder

½ tsp ground cinnamon

1 cooking apple, peeled, cored and
    cut into ribbons using a vegetable
    peeler

1½ tbsp natural yogurt, to serve

Apple & Ricotta Tarts

Serves: 2

Preparation time:
15 minutes

Cooking time:
20 minutes

Here's a recipe that you are sure to love because it is so versatile, it works amazingly with almost any fruit. Plus, let's be honest, filo pastry makes an interesting addition to almost any dish.

1   Preheat the oven to 200°C/400°F/gas 6 and line a baking tray with baking paper.

2   Cut 1 sheet of filo pastry into quarters and place a quarter in the baking tray. Spray lightly with low-calorie oil spray, put the next quarter on top, then repeat with the other pieces. Repeat this process to create 2 pastry beds.

3   Mix together the ricotta, vanilla extract, stevia powder and cinnamon in a bowl. Smooth this on top of the pastry beds, then lay the apple ribbons evenly on top. Bake for about 20 minutes until the filo pastry is crisp at the edges and the apple is soft. Serve warm with a spoonful of yogurt.

NUTRITION NOTES
PER SERVING
••••••••••••••••••
• Calories: 227kcals
• Fat: 8g
• Carbohydrates: 31g

2 cooking apples, peeled, cored and
    thinly sliced
2 tsp lemon juice
2 tsp stevia powder

2 tsp ground cinnamon
35g/1¼oz/⅓ cup rolled oats
1 tbsp wholemeal flour
2 tbsp flaked almonds

1 tsp freshly grated nutmeg
1 tsp almond extract
1 tbsp butter
1½ tbsp natural yogurt, to serve

Almond Apple Crumble

Serves: 2

Preparation time:
10 minutes

Cooking time:
35 minutes

A true family favourite, I like to indulge in a bowl of crumble on a lazy Sunday evening on the sofa. And just because this is a really healthy version of a traditional crumble, don't worry – you won't be disappointed because it tastes as good as it looks (see pages 142–43). Try it as your weekend indulgence.

1   Preheat the oven to 180°C/350°F/gas 4. Put the apple slices in a bowl, sprinkle with the lemon juice, stevia powder and cinnamon and toss to coat the apples. Put them in the bottom of a small baking dish.

2   Mix together the oats, flour, almonds, nutmeg and almond extract in a bowl. Add the butter and rub in with your fingertips until the mixture resembles coarse breadcrumbs. Spoon over the apples, then bake for about 35 minutes, or until the top is golden and crisp. Serve warm with a spoonful of yogurt on the top.

NUTRITION NOTES
PER SERVING
....
• Calories: 249kcals
• Fat: 13g
• Carbohydrates: 29g

low-calorie cooking oil spray

2 sheets of filo pastry

2 tbsp flaked almonds

2 large sticks of rhubarb, chopped

1 tsp ground cinnamon, plus extra
   for sprinkling

2 tsp stevia powder

2 tbsp Greek yogurt

agave nectar, to taste

Rhubarb Filo Cup with Cinnamon & Greek Yogurt

Serves: 2

Preparation time:
15 minutes

Cooking time:
15 minutes

When rhubarb is in season, it is a staple in my household, as I just love the sticky, sweet and sour flavours you get when you serve it hot with cold yogurt. You may be surprised at how pretty this simple dessert looks once prepared – it is almost too good to eat … but not quite!

1 Preheat the oven to 180°C/350°F/gas 4 and lightly mist two sections of a deep muffin tin with low-calorie oil spray. Lay the sheets of filo pastry on a chopping board and lightly mist both sides with the spray, then cut each one into 4 squares. Press one of the squares into the prepared muffin tin to create a cup shape, then lay another 3 squares of filo pastry over the top to create a layered cup. Repeat with the remaining filo pastry squares to make 2 layered cups. Bake for 10–15 minutes until golden and crisp.

2 Meanwhile, heat a heavy-based frying pan over a medium heat. Add the almonds and cook for 2–3 minutes, stirring continuously, until lightly browned. Remove them from the pan immediately so they don't over-brown.

3 Put the rhubarb, cinnamon, stevia powder and 120ml/3¾fl oz/scant ½ cup of water in a non-stick saucepan over a medium heat. Cover with a lid and cook for about 5 minutes, stirring frequently, until softened and pulpy, adding more water if the mixture becomes too dry.

4 Remove the filo cups from the muffin tin and transfer to a plate. Evenly spoon the rhubarb filling into each cup and top each one with the yogurt and toasted almonds. Drizzle with agave nectar, sprinkle with a little cinnamon and serve hot.

NUTRITION NOTES
PER SERVING
• • • • • • • • • • • • • • • •
• Calories: 126kcals
• Fat: 4g
• Carbohydrates: 20g

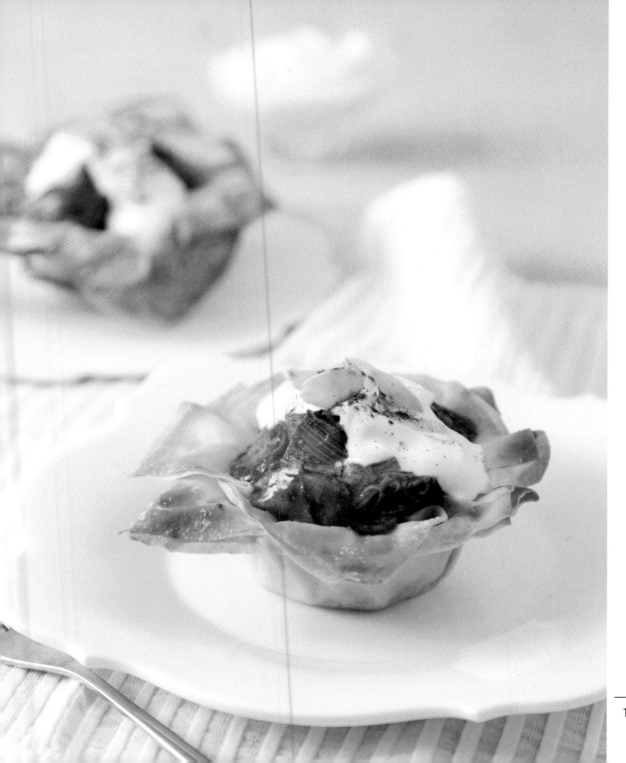

½ banana, mashed

25g/1oz/¼ cup rolled oats

2 tsp almond extract

1 tsp stevia powder

1 egg white

a pinch of ground cinnamon, plus
extra for sprinkling

50g/1¾oz/½ cup pecan nuts, finely
chopped

2 large peaches, halved and pitted

1½ tbsp natural yogurt, to serve

Baked Pecan-Stuffed Peaches

Serves: 2

Preparation time:
10 minutes

Cooking time:
20 minutes

This is a great summer dessert as it is best made when peaches are in season and full of flavour and goodness. Served hot or cold, the baking brings out the natural flavours and sweetness of the fruit. You can try it with nectarines, too.

1 Preheat the oven to 180°C/350°F/gas 4. In a bowl, mix together the banana, oats, almond extract, stevia powder, egg white, cinnamon and pecans.

2 Put the peach halves, cut-sides up, in a baking dish. Sprinkle with the oat mixture and bake for about 20 minutes, or until soft and slightly golden on top.

3 Sprinkle with a little more cinnamon and serve warm or cold with a dollop of yogurt on top or served separately.

NUTRITION NOTES
PER SERVING
• • • • • • • • • • • • • • • •
• Calories: 360kcals
• Fat: 23g
• Carbohydrates: 35g

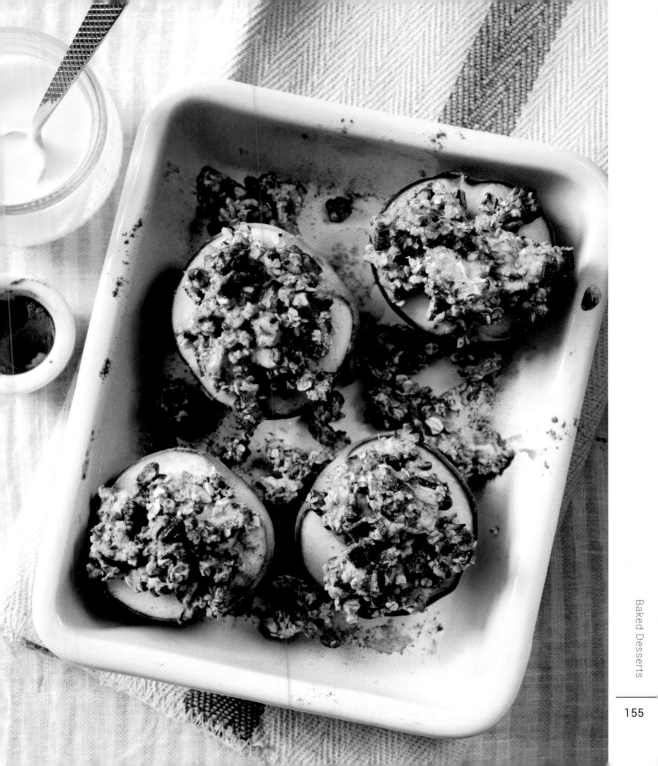

FOR THE BASE

low-calorie cooking oil spray

15g/½oz/scant ¼ cup ground
    almonds

4 oat cakes

½ tsp freshly grated nutmeg

1 tsp agave nectar

1 tbsp butter

FOR THE FILLING

1 gelatine leaf

6 strawberries, hulled

2 tbsp cream cheese

2 tsp natural yogurt

1 tsp agave nectar

1 tsp vanilla extract

Mini Strawberry Cheesecakes

Serves: 2

Preparation time:
25 minutes, plus
1 hour chilling

Cooking time:
5 minutes

These little treats are great because they are both healthy and have a low GI, which means they release their energy slowly into the body. They are deliciously fresh and creamy with a crumbly, chewy base.

1   Lightly mist two sections of a deep muffin tin with low-calorie oil spray.

2   Put the gelatine in a small bowl, just cover with cold water and leave to soak for 5 minutes. Transfer the gelatine to a small saucepan over a low heat and leave to melt for about 1 minute.

3   Meanwhile, put the ground almonds, oat cakes, nutmeg and agave nectar in a blender or food processor and blend to form crumbs, then transfer to a bowl. Put the butter into a small saucepan over a low heat until melted, then stir into the crumb mixture. Spoon the mixture into the prepared tins and flatten down with the back of a spoon.

4   Blend the strawberries in a blender or food processor until liquid, then add the cream cheese, yogurt, agave nectar and vanilla extract and stir together well. Finally, stir in the gelatine and mix thoroughly. Spoon over the biscuit bases and chill for at least 1 hour before serving.

NUTRITION NOTES
PER SERVING
••••••••••••••••••
• Calories: 374kcals
• Fat: 23g
• Carbohydrates: 25g

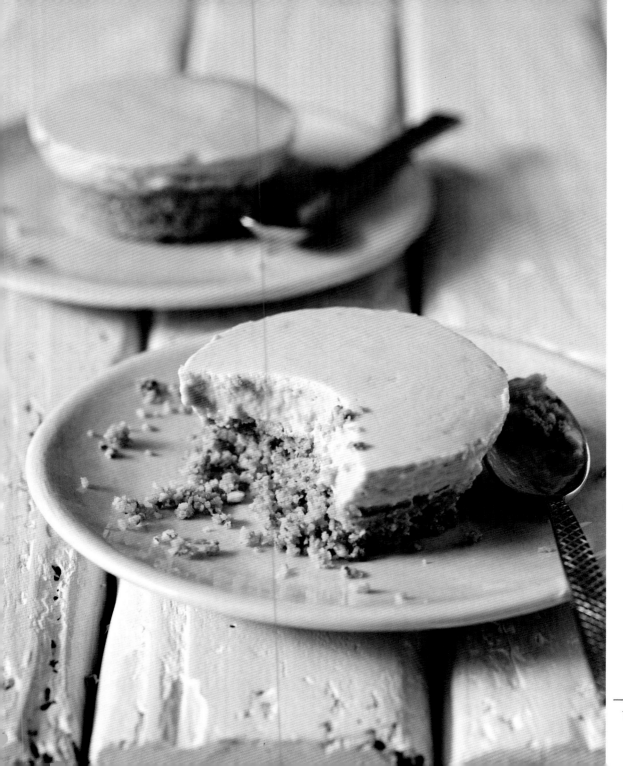

2 egg whites

2 tbsp unsweetened desiccated
   coconut

7 walnuts, finely chopped

1 tsp stevia powder

¼ tsp cream of tartar

½ tsp vanilla extract

40g/1½oz dark chocolate, 70% cocoa
   solids, broken into pieces

Chocolate Walnut Macaroons

Serves: 2

Preparation time:
20 minutes, plus
1 hour chilling

Cooking time:
20 minutes

These may be old-fashioned but who cares? They are still one of the most delicious desserts as far as I'm concerned. Who can resist that crisp outer layer hiding the meltingly soft, chewy centre?

1 Preheat the oven to 170°C/325°F/gas 3 and line a baking tray with baking paper. In a large bowl, whisk the egg whites until light and frothy. Add the coconut, walnuts, stevia powder, cream of tartar and vanilla extract. Use a spatula to gently fold the mixture together until it has all blended evenly. Shape the mixture into 2 large macaroons on the prepared baking tray. Bake for about 20 minutes until firm.

2 Meanwhile, put the chocolate in a large heatproof bowl and rest it over a pan of gently simmering water, making sure that the bottom of the bowl does not touch the water. Heat, stirring occasionally, until the chocolate has melted. Remove the pan from the heat.

3 Transfer the macaroons to a wire rack, then use a spoon to drizzle the melted chocolate over the top. Leave to finish cooling, then chill in the fridge for at least 1 hour before serving.

NUTRITION NOTES
PER SERVING
• • • • • • • • • • • • • • • •
• Calories: 328kcals
• Fat: 28g
• Carbohydrates: 12g

Dessert Recipes